THE HUMOROUS HERBALIST

Laurel Dewey

Cover Design & Illustrations
Jack Jones

The Humorous Herbalist
Glenwood Springs, Colorado

10 9 8 7 6 5 4 3 2

ISBN 1-884820-23-9

Safe Goods
P. O. Box 36
East Canaan, CT 06024

(860) 824-5301

Manufactured in the United States of America.

This book is dedicated to
Mom & Dad
& Granny
For their encouragement
support
humor
&
sage advice

Thanks to Pat Noel at Carbondale, Colorado's *Valley Journal* for saying "yes" to the first "Humorous Herbalist" column. You helped get this whole thing started.

CONTENTS

Introduction 1

An Herb is an Herb is a Healer? 6

Herbs, Herbs, Herbs 10

Are You Ready For Arnica? 11

Calendula— The Mighty Marigold with Moxie! 15

Cascara Sagrada— A Moving Experience..................................... 20

Catnip— The Paws That Refreshes 24

Cayenne— It's Not Just For Breakfast Anymore.......................... 28

I'd Walk a Mile for Some Chamomile 35

Comfrey—A Bone-ified Herbal Healer.. 41

Dandelion—A Lifesaver for Your Liver.. 47

Dong Quai For Me... 52

Echinacea—The Lymphomaniac Herb 58

Be Kind to Your Elder.. 64

You can Breathe with Eucalyptus!... 68

Gads! It's Garlic!... 73

You Don't Have to be Fred to Like Ginger! 80

Ginseng May Put the Zing Back in Your Spring!......................... 86

Hops—the Beer-less Brew to Snooze On 92

Juniper—Just Say Go! 97

Lavender— It's Siesta Time! 102

Licorice— a Beaut of a Root... 107

Parsley—the Garnish with Gusto.. 112

The Power's in the Peppermint.. 117

Plantain & Simple... 123

Rally 'Round Red Raspberry Leaf... 128

St. John's Wort—the Wound-Healing Herb with the Weird Name 133

White Willow—Barking up the Headache Tree............................. 140

The Herbal Bath Hath What It Takes!... 146

Putting Your Foot in the Right Concoction................................... 154

15 Really Good Questions People Ask About Herbs...................... 159

How To Make Your Own Herbal First Aid Kit.............................. 168

Quick & Easy Reference Chart for Common Ailments.................. 171

How to Make Herbal Stuff.. 184

Bibliography & Reference... 194

Index 201

INTRODUCTION

The Humorous Herbalist was born—first as a national syndicated newspaper column and now as the book you hold in your hand.

Why did I write this book? Libraries are filled with books on herbs. However, I know from personal experience that most of them are not fun to read. I wanted to change that, to write an herb book that was informative, humorous and a viable reference guide. A book that said "Go on. Read me. You'll like me."

For me, natural medicine has always been well, natural. I didn't "get into it"—rather, I grew up with it. My mother believed in natural remedies and used them on countless occasions. When I'd fall and bruise my knee, *homeopathic* arnica was the stuff that would help the bruise. If I burned my finger, calendula ointment was the proven remedy. And when the common cold caught me, several servings of homemade chicken soup with fresh garlic and onions was the way to get well.

I can honestly say that most of the childhood illnesses I had were treated with either herbs or homeopathy. And to this day, I continue to use natural medicine first as a preventative against illness as well as a healing helper.

I don't, however, *depend* upon herbs to get me through each and every day. Even on the preventative front, about the only herb I use on a semi-regular basis is garlic.

On the practical side, there are various reasons why a person shouldn't become totally dependent upon herbs. Herbs are medicine in the purist form. And just like any medicine, complete dependency is not always healthy. In addition, continual intake of many herbs can produce toxicity within the body. The body becomes so saturated with an herb or herbal formula that it starts to ignore the original purpose of the herb. When your body reaches this particular point, the herb is unable to accomplish its purpose and it turns on the body. It does this by creating toxicity. If you take one herb (or formula) for too long, you can become in a sense, immune to the herb's effectiveness. As always, there are herbs which are an exception to this rule.

It's all about *balance*. When one is out of balance—physically, mentally or even spiritually—the body will become open to disease. Natural medicine practitioners are fond of saying, one should think of disease as "dis-ease" within the body. The goal of natural therapies is to bring the body back into center. Once it's there, you simply need to *maintain* that balance.

Famous herbalist, Dr. John R. Christopher, believed that an herb should be taken for six days, rest one day without it, then continue again for six days. He felt this routine should continue for three to six weeks. After that, STOP for one to three weeks and allow the body to utilize what it has been given, flush out what it doesn't need, realign itself and then adjust itself to its new alignment. Once all that takes place, you can see how you feel and continue on the six day on one day off cycle or simply use the herb two to three times a week as a maintenance program. *(Note: There are herbs which should not be taken daily for longer than three weeks at a time because of their tendency to build up extreme toxicity within the body and/or exacerbate chronic physical conditions within the body—such as high blood pressure or low blood sugar. Before taking ANY herb, read as much about it as possible.)*

◊ ◊ ◊

The difference between the way herbs work inside the body vs. drug therapy is that herbs *support* the body's natural defenses which help to trigger the healing process. While they can kill infection, drugs tend to *suppress* symptoms, making it more difficult for the body's natural defenses to kick in. After long-term use of antibiotics and over-the-counter medication, the body becomes extremely toxic. It then becomes harder for the body to create any defense mechanism which can fight against disease.

For those of you who are new to herbs and have spent much of your life using chemical medicines, I strongly suggest you enter into this different way of life gradually. *(This does not apply if you have been taking daily prescriptions for chronic health problems. Never eliminate doctor-prescribed medications and replace them with herbs or any other natural treatments without first checking with your doctor.)* For the rest of the readers who are not committed to a daily, doctor-prescribed prescription, here is some food for thought. Instead of eliminating chemical medications (such as cold and flu antibiotics or over-the-counter sinus and cough medications), try simply reducing the *amount* of chemical treatment while incorporating an herbal tea, tincture or capsule into your regimen. Over time, continue to cut back on chemical medications and introduce more natural remedies into your body.

I have seen too many people quit antibiotics and over-the-counter flu remedies cold turkey in an attempt to become overnight herb converts. What usually happens is their body has no idea what to do with the herbs because it has been battling the synthetic pills and potions. Continual use of non-natural medications for long periods of time has a cumulative effect on the body and, over time, suppresses the body's natural immune system.

When I refer to the use of chemical medications, I mean continual (monthly, daily, weekly) dependence upon *un*-natural treatments to "cure" everything from a headache to a stomach ache. The result of *excessive* synthetic medication is a very toxic system. That built up toxicity forces your body to work harder every time you get sick.

Because of this, it can be difficult to go from *un*-natural to natural medicine at once. After years of suppressing colds, flu and the like with chemical medications, your body has become accustomed to receiving the drugs and *expects* to ingest them whenever it becomes ill. But, never fear, your body will gradually "re-learn" what to do with the herbs and soon adapt to this gentler, less toxic approach to health.

◊ ◊ ◊

If you are serious about turning your life around and tackling your pains and ailments with natural medicine, it would be sensible to first make an appointment with a qualified and respected holistic doctor who can give you a general physical examination. The doctor may suggest you do a detoxifying cleanse over a period of weeks to release the built up toxicity in your body. Virtually *nothing* can be treated if your body is still fighting the effects of chemical toxicity. One doesn't need to go to a doctor to detoxify the body. However, depending upon how severe your *accumulated* problems are, it can be a tricky process. If you detoxify too quickly, fevers can often be the result as well as excessive perspiration, headaches, joint pain, dizziness and painful bowel cramps. These symptoms are all a result of releasing too much toxic poison at once. (Herbalists like to call this response a "healing crisis"). A good holistic doctor can "pace" the detox process and work to avoid any unnecessary or uncomfortable consequences.

◊ ◊ ◊

If you decide to go with a natural approach using herbs, remember the following saying, "Treat the *source* of the illness NOT the *symptom* of the illness." *This is the key to all healing.*

Finding that *source* is not always easy. I'm a big believer in the mind/body connection and feel that the *source* for many minor to chronic ailments can stem from a deeper, more emotional root. Some natural practitioners claim that every single ailment starts in the emotional body before it attacks the physical. No matter what you believe, the resulting pain and discomfort manifests in the physical body and something needs to be done.

If that "something" happens to be herbs, you've come to the right book. And to answer the question, "Why did I write this book?" I can say simply this: I know herbs work. I know herbs can be a better, safer, healthier way to heal the body. When you really "get into" all the flowers, roots, leaves and barks, it's a fascinating journey. And I bet that you'll find yourself saying at least once, "I didn't know one little plant could do *that!*"

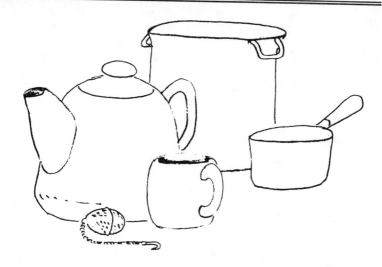

Important
When you are making your teas,
please **DO NOT** use aluminum or cast iron pots.

The aluminum and iron can alter the ability of the herb to work as a medicinal agent. Use a good grade of stainless steel (one that is not made partly with aluminum) or pyrex. Enamel pans are fine, however make sure there are no chips or cracks and that the pot is fully enamel-covered.

In addition, while it is not imperative to your good health, it is best to use *distilled* water when making all medicinal herb teas. When it comes in contact with an herb, distilled water has a tendency to "suck" more of the nutrients out of the plant than tap water. Also, because distilled water is more "purified" than tap water, it is unlikely to conflict with the natural chemical balance within each plant.

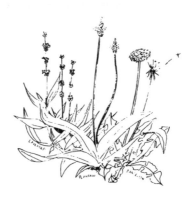

AN HERB IS AN HERB IS A HEALER?

Herbs are a lot like people. Some can help you and some can harm you. When you use them properly—which means using an herb in correct amounts and for the reasons it is meant for—that latter part won't happen.

Whether you call them herbs or 'erbs, it doesn't matter. Most folks couldn't even begin to pronounce their Latin names. Perhaps that's why early herbalists in the 17th century decided to give herbs names that seemed appropriate based entirely on their look and color. Odd names such as devil's claw, horsetail, bladderwrack, lungwort, lady's slipper, heal all, and my personal favorite, wahoo, were handed out to herbs according to what the herb *might* be able to cure. For example, some fellow looked at lungwort herb and said "You know, those specks on that leaf look a heck of a lot like a pair of lungs. How 'bout we say it's good for the lungs." Well, it just so happens that lungwort *is* one herb that is used for bronchial conditions. But an herb such as bladderwrack is not for bladder complaints. And the herb wahoo *doesn't* necessarily make one want to "yippee."

Still, those early herbalists pressed on, experimenting on each other with wild herbs, intent on trying to find the perfect match between the ailment and the herb that would help or even cure the condition. They had a few hits, a lot of misses and many final words probably were "I thought you said that root would make me feel *better*."

But through time, patience and considerable study, the perfect matches were found. For hundreds of years, nature's backyard provided thousands of families with everything they needed throughout their life to bring down a fever, fight infection, mend a broken bone and soothe the spirit.

Fast forward to the present day and to many people, the idea of foraging in the forest for a healing plant ranks right up there with throwing salt over your shoulder to ensure good luck. People want drugs and they want them NOW! Yet, while herbs may not have the synthesized, stark potency of the average antibiotic, many are able to work more effectively than some antibiotics because they help the body to naturally fight off the illness while fully supporting it in the process. That's not to say that herbs are perfect and work every time you take them. Nor are antibiotics evil little monsters that mess you up for life. The irony is that about 54% of today's most sought after drugs are derived from an herb which has been unceremoniously stripped of all its balancing agents, reduced to a single active part, and synthetically converted into very potent medication. For example, quinine comes from the Peruvian "fever tree" (cinchona), aspirin was born out of white willow bark, and digitalis is the synthetic drug partly extracted from the foxglove plant. All these drugs are helpful and can relieve pain and suffering. But most herbalists will agree that when you extract only a section of a plant, flower, or tree bark, and discard the rest, you are robbing both plant and patient of the herb in its true, natural, healing form. Over time, the synthetic result may deplete your body of its ability to fight off infection.

If you make the decision to take the natural approach and convert your body into an herbal haven, *always* consider the following criteria very carefully:

- Read everything you can about the herbs you want to take—and I don't just mean the handful of words on the back of the herb box! Don't be fooled into believing that all herbs are just wimpy little plants with no punch. Herbs *can* be powerful medicine. For example, some herbs which stimulate the nervous system can sometimes create agitation which could keep you up at night. Others may work on the intestine and colon which might produce diarrhea with overuse.
- Find out when you should take the herbs and most importantly, when you should *not* take them. Some herbs have particular

qualities which can cause adverse effects in people with specific conditions. Some of these conditions are:

- Pregnancy
- Heart problems
- High/low blood pressure
- High/low/irregular blood sugar (i.e., diabetes)
- Any chronic conditions which need regular medical supervision and/or prescriptions.

If you have any of the above, it does not mean you can't take herbs. BUT you need to be fully aware of how the herb reacts in the body. Pregnant women, especially, need to be very careful since many herbs stimulate the uterus. There are some herbs that are beneficial to women during certain periods in pregnancy. However, I highly recommend that if you are pregnant, you consult a qualified holistic doctor who can suggest specific "support" herbs based upon your previous medical history.

Herbology isn't so much complicated as it is full of details. There are many variables that need to be considered before delving into an herbal lifestyle.

- Some herbs are considered highly toxic. About 1% can kill you. Jimson weed, for example, can produce hellish hallucinations and even death. Black, green or fetid hellebore could also hasten your departure. And deadly nightshade wasn't given its name simply for the shock value—the berries are poison. Herbal books call such herbs "restricted," which means that one should not take the herb at all or limit their dosage *but do this only under a holistic practitioner's care.*

In relation to this, I'm not a big advocate of going out in the woods and picking wild herbs for internal consumption unless you or someone you are with is skilled in this pursuit. Too many plants look alike and you risk not only picking the wrong plant but a toxic one as well! For example, a plant called "dog poison" looks very much like wild parsley. (In fact, the folk name for dog poison is "fool's-parsley.") By all accounts, "dog poison" is dead poison and a few mouthfuls can be fatal.

Commercial preparations are best in lieu of growing the herbs yourself. However, it *does* matter how you cultivate the plants and prepare the soil. Poor soil often yields weak, spindly plants that don't retain as much nutritional value. And spraying chemical pesticides over your medicinal herbs is like dipping a vitamin in gasoline before ingesting. Since one usually takes medicinal herbs for their natural, healing benefits, it doesn't make much sense to treat the herb with un-natural sprays that can soak clear through to the root! It is important to remember this fact if you decide to purchase herbs from a local herb farm. Find out how the plants are grown and if they use chemical or organic pest deterrents.

- Know your body's tolerance and weaknesses. Everyone's chemistry is unique and one herb might be perfect for one person and harmful to another. Persons who have depended upon antibiotics most of their life might find switching to herbology difficult at first. The body could fight against the plants and for awhile you may need to continue with small amounts of an antibiotic.

- At first it's best not to mix different herbs together at home until you learn about the cause and effect of each one as well as how they chemically inter-relate. Herbal formulas can work wonders since one is benefiting from the combined effect of each plant as it interacts with the others. While homemade formulas may indeed work, commercial herbal formulas are usually more dependable since they are carefully measured and combined.

When seeking out an herbal supplement, it's a good idea to find a company that has been in the business for a long time and has a good reputation. If you start to get into herbal medicine, you'll begin to see the same brand names in many stores. Major labels don't always equal major quality, though, so ask around, find out what brands other people use and then make a decision.

Lately, many companies have started using what they call "guaranteed potency" herbs. It means that the herbal chemist has taken the time to include consistent levels of the herb's potent medicinal center which "guarantees" a more active supplement. In essence, with "guaranteed potency" herbs, you're getting more bang for your buck.

- Most importantly, don't throw your doctor's phone number away. Just because you have decided to "go natural" doesn't mean traditional medicine has to go out the door. To get the best of both worlds, it would be most advantageous to find a medical doctor who has a profound interest and respect for alternative medicine.

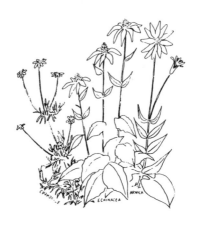

HERBS, HERBS, HERBS

I picked 25 herbs to include in this book. That wasn't easy since there are well over 300,000. I selected the following herbs for various reasons. First, many are well known—such as chamomile and peppermint. However, chamomile is not just a nice "sleepy time" tea and peppermint is not just a good tasting after-dinner beverage. So, chances are you'll learn something new.

Secondly, I wanted to include a wide range of herbs that covered everything from the common cold to the common headache. What 25 herbs would I choose if I were stranded on a deserted island. Hopefully, after reading about the individual herbs, you will want to buy a couple of them to keep in your cupboard. Maybe you'll want to go all out and buy an ounce of each herb mentioned just in case *you* find yourself on a deserted island.

Thirdly, I chose 25 herbs that are easy to find in any health/herb store, no matter where you live. I'll leave the exotic, hard-to-find jungle herbs for someone else.

At the top of each herbal chapter, you'll find the herb's Latin name, the medicinal parts of the plant and in what forms the herb is taken. Within each chapter, I've placed the uses for each herb in **bold lettering** as well as the cautions that need to be addressed.

So, relax and enjoy your trip down herbal lane.

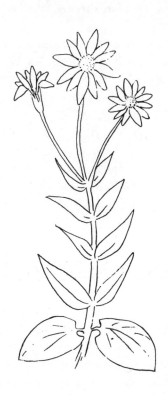

ARE YOU READY FOR ARNICA?

Latin name: *Arnica montana*
Medicinal parts: flowers, roots
Forms: tea bath, tincture, ointment
(all externally only!)
For internal use, only use homeopathic arnica

Ah, bruises. Nature's little tattoos to show the world that you fell down, bumped into something or ran into the wall. Your generic bruises come in the standard black and blue, but the exotic brands—usually courtesy of dramatic accidents—take on a bright spectrum of animated colors that would make Walt Disney jealous.

Most bruises don't require more than a casual glance. But others—especially those that occur during post-surgery or when you have had a serious accident—need special attention. And catch this:

there is an herb called arnica that tackles this battle of the **bruises.** Arnica is in the same family as calendula (see the next chapter), but unlike calendula, it does its herbal work externally rather than internally. **This is important because taking arnica HERB internally can be fatal.** And yet externally, it can be the one herb you reach for whenever you fall down and go boom.

There are four ways to use arnica: in a tincture, an ointment, a tea bath or internally only in its homeopathic tablet form. Homeopathic arnica is the only form in which you can take arnica internally. I'm not trying to confuse you when I say this, but the homeopathic arnica is different than the herb. The homeopathic can be taken orally because the homeopathic tablet goes through a different tincturing process that enables the herb to be safely used internally. Suffice to say that I highly recommend keeping a bottle of homeopathic arnica (either 6x or 30x) in your purse and/or glove compartment.

I grew up with arnica in both its homeopathic and tincture form. Being the naive kid that I was, I figured everyone had arnica tucked away in their medicine chest. When the girl down the block hit her head and a bump formed, I innocently said, "Just take arnica tablets and it'll go away." Needless to say, I was considered a tad weird in my youth.

Arnica, in its homeopathic form, is the very first thing you should reach for when you or someone else has had any type of **shock or trauma to the body that could result in bruising or inflammation.** With homeopathic arnica, the motto is "the sooner the better" for quick results. Once, I saw a neighbor slip on the icy pavement in front of her house. She banged her shoulder and within minutes, a bruise was forming under her skin. She was due to leave the next day on a long road trip and was worried she'd have to cancel. I quickly suggested homeopathic arnica and she took nine tablets (three right away, and three one and two hours later). She looked kind of leery of the idea, as if she were simply taking the tablets to pacify me. But the next morning, she was at my door smiling before taking off in her car, saying she could not believe how good she felt. There was no bruising and only slight swelling.

If it's possible, homeopathic arnica should be taken on an empty stomach. As I said before, look for the 6x or 30x potency which will be written on the label of the bottle (6x is for children under 12

years old and 30x is for adults.) Homeopathic arnica is also dandy
to have on hand for toddlers when they start toddling. They are
bound to take some minor falls which can result in bumping their
bodies into furniture, walls and pavements. All of this can, of
course, cause painful bruises and miserable kids. For toddlers,
homeopathic arnica in a potency of 3x can be a lifesaver. Usually,
they'll only need one 3x tablet after the mishap and then one several
hours later. Don't forget, for homeopathic arnica to be most
effective, it needs to be given to the child immediately. The tiny
tablets (which are more like little pellets) can be easily administered
because they are in a fast-dissolving suc lac base.

Homeopathic arnica has helped me avoid bruises of all types—
even those which might occur. For instance, before I had four
impacted wisdom teeth extracted, the oral surgeon told me to expect
to look like a raccoon after surgery due to the heavy bruising that
would form around my eyes. "The roots on these babies are deep,"
he explained with an air of excitement. "As deep as the roots on an
oak tree. There is no way you are going to avoid major bruising and
swelling. See you tomorrow!"

I started taking homeopathic arnica tablets (30x) the day before
surgery—about two every four hours. The next morning, I had
those suckers yanked out of my jaw and as soon as I stopped
spitting up blood, I continued to take homeopathic arnica—this time,
about two every hour for the first day. I NEVER, I say NEVER,
experienced one bruise or even the slightest puff or swelling.
Doubters will say I was an exception to the bruising rule. Herbalists
and homeopaths will say otherwise.

The other forms of arnica—the tincture, ointment and tea bath—
are all used externally. The tincture is probably the most widely used
external form of the herb. And once again, **bruising or swelling**
are the signposts for using arnica tincture.

Arnica tincture—made from a base of arnica flowers and pure
grain alcohol that ranges between 80 and 100 proof—can be drying
or cause a burning sensation on sensitive skin. Because of this, it's
always best to dilute the tincture with water. **The only caution
here is that arnica tincture cannot be used on broken or
bleeding skin**. The high alcohol content can blister and burn an
open wound. In addition, arnica has been known to prevent blood
from clotting. **This caution also applies to arnica ointment.**

A bottle of arnica tincture is a first aid necessity if you or someone you know **sprains** their wrist, finger or ankle. The first thing to do is soak a cotton pad in arnica tincture and tape it directly to the sprain. Remember, with arnica, the sooner you can administer it, the sooner the healing will begin. After applying the arnica tincture, two to three homeopathic arnica tablets can be taken to bolster the anti-inflammation/anti-bruising effect. This practice should never replace seeing a doctor. It simply is a buffer against unnecessary pain and swelling that can inhibit the healing process.

One of the lesser known uses for arnica tincture is as an external treatment for **TMJ**. One herbalist friend of mine swears that when he soaks a cotton ball in arnica tincture and then gently strokes the jaw bone area with the cotton ball, the TMJ discomfort is greatly reduced. If you or someone you know suffers from TMJ, you've got nothing to lose by trying this simple external treatment.

Except for **TMJ**, arnica ointment can be used for all the same reasons you would use the tincture. The ointment also works as a topical treatment whenever you get **insect bites,** helping to disinfect the bite and speed the healing process.

An arnica tea bath works as a gentle wash to soothe **strains and sprains**. You can either use the tea in the bathtub or in a pail as a soothing soak for feet, hands or elbows. For the bath, boil four quarts of water. Turn off the flame and gently stir in two cups of dried arnica flowers. Let the herbs steep like a big tea for 20 minutes. Strain and pour into a hot tub and soak your weary limbs for up to 30 minutes.

As a foot bath, you'll only need one cup of dried arnica flowers. You also don't need to strain the arnica flowers since you don't have to worry about clogging drains in a bucket. Soak your feet as long as the water stays warm. This "bucket-bath" works well for people who, because of their injury, may have trouble getting in and out of a tub. A cold water foot bath with arnica tea makes a wonderful anti-inflammatory soak for **sprained ankles**. Make the mixture as mentioned above, but set it aside to cool. (To speed the cooling process, add ice cubes to the tea.) Soak the sprained ankle from twenty minutes to two hours in the foot bath. The combination of cold water and arnica flowers works wonders to reduce puffiness and pain.

Time and time again, I've seen arnica in all its many forms, stop the painful results of a serious injury and alleviate unnecessary suffering after surgery.

You can bet I never leave home without it.

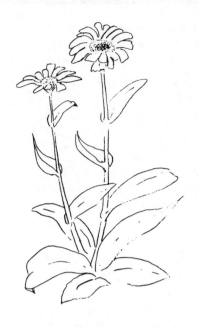

CALENDULA—
THE MIGHTY.
MARIGOLD
WITH MOXIE!

Latin name: *Calendula officinalis*
Medicinal parts: leaves, flowers
Forms: tea, ointment, tincture, oil extraction

When other kids scraped their knees, they'd reach for Bactine or Iodine. When I found myself in that predicament, my mother applied calendula ointment. I thought Bactine smelled like gasoline and Iodine made skin look like it was bleeding rust. Calendula ointment, on the other hand, was clean, lightly scented and didn't hurt or sting.

Oh, and it worked—better than those other drug store specials. When I was young, calendula ointment was an oddity. Today, calendula is the base or main ingredient in many skin products—ranging from skin lotions to eye creams.

While I can't recommend using the merry marigold in place of The Weather Channel, I can highly endorse its healing ability.

Calendula (pronounced "ka-*len*-ju-la" *not* "*kal*-en-du-la" as some folks have been known to say) is considered a reliable remedy for almost every problem that has to do with the skin. Herbalists have been using it for ages. During World War I, it was physicians who were sold on the marigold's healing effects. They noticed that tinctures and ointments made of pure marigold flowers did a bang up job on putrid wounds. Not only did calendula work as a fast-acting antiseptic, it also sped up the healing time. Ironically, this has a lot to do with its high content of *natural* iodine. Yes, the common marigold may look like just another "pretty flower," but hidden within those petals are **strong antiseptic, anti-fungal and anti-inflammatory properties**.

Calendula is used in four forms: tea, ointment, tincture and oil. To give you an overview of what calendula in its different incarnations can do, I'll start with the ointment since I feel it has the most uses.

The Ointment—Primarily, I've always turned to the ointment for quick relief from **minor burns** caused by the sun or the stove, as well as **minor scratches and scrapes.** Besides taking the heat out of the burn, calendula ointment soaks through the layers of skin to start the healing process. Many times when I've used calendula ointment on a burn, I've never had to worry about the accompanying blister that usually appears within a day. Also, the ointment, which is a **powerful anti-inflammatory**, allows the scrape or burn to heal without leaving any scar.

Speaking of **scars**, I have first hand experience with the ointment's ability to reduce and even "dissolve" old scars that didn't heal correctly. This won't happen overnight, but by rubbing in a small amount of the ointment over stubborn scars for a period of 10-16 weeks, I was able to get rid of them permanently.

Use the ointment as a topical treatment whenever you have any kind of **skin problem, including dry eczema.** The ointment is also excellent for **nursing mothers** who suffer from **sore nipples**. If the ointment is applied sparingly after each feeding, the pain and inflammation can be reduced within days.

The ointment is great for **cracked, dry skin** as long as you use it on a semi-regular basis. When the cold weather arrives, **chapped or severely cracked lips** are sure to follow. I have truly found that calendula ointment is *the* most effective chapped lip treatment. Best of all, it never leaves any sticky residue. And you don't have to keep reapplying it every hour because it soaks in cleanly, leaving a top layer of moisture protection.

There have been cases where the ointment has also helped reduce **varicose veins.** (Of course, diet, exercise and elevating one's feet at least 15 minutes a day, are all part of the plan when treating this painful problem). It's best to apply a thick coat of the ointment morning and night, taking care to rub it gently into your skin. It may take several months before you see any change. I have heard of everything from a 10-50% reduction in pain.

If you get **scabs** in your nose, calendula ointment applied lightly over the area will help to soften them and discourage any further outbreaks. For this reason, calendula ointment is a good treatment for **impetigo**.

Amazingly, the ointment also does double duty to prevent as well as treat **bedsores**. The skin is left extremely soft and the patient eternally grateful.

The Tincture—Because most tinctures have an alcohol base, there is a natural drying aspect to them. Couple calendula's ability to heal the skin, and the tincture works as an excellent remedy for **cold sores and canker sores.** For **cold sores**, soak a cotton ball in the tincture. Depending upon your sensitivity to the alcohol, either hold it firmly on the cold sore or lightly dab the area. The same applies for **canker sores**. At the first "feel" of a canker sore, I apply a heavily moistened cotton ball of calendula tincture on the area and hold it in place for as long as three minutes. Often, I will first soak the cotton ball in cold water before pouring the tincture into it. I do this only because sometimes if the alcohol content is too high in the tincture, you can literally pull a thin layer of skin off your mouth. As you hold the tincture-soaked cotton ball in place, there may be a slight sting and your eyes might tear up, but I assure you it's not painful—just "pulling" as the tincture immediately starts drawing out the fire inside the sore. I've seen this work literally overnight to reduce or even eliminate the canker sore.

Calendula tincture also is handy to have around for minor cuts and scrapes. Not only does it work to **stop bleeding**, it also helps speed healing. Unlike arnica tincture, you can pour the tincture undiluted into an open, bleeding wound or mix 6-10 drops of the tincture in a tablespoon of warm water and pour that over the wound. Many folks have claimed that by repeating this process several times each day, the wound is almost fully healed within three days—and without leaving any scars.

The tincture can be taken internally for the same reasons one would drink the tea. (See the section on calendula tea for specific ailments). The usual tincture dosage is 8-10 drops in 8 oz. of hot water.

The Oil—While the healing emollients are present in calendula oil, it doesn't always have the staying power of the ointment which tends to "stick" to the skin better. However, you can use calendula oil as a topical skin treatment just like you would the ointment. Many mothers prefer the oil to the ointment when it comes to **diaper rash** since the oil soaks into the baby's skin with no greasy top coat. Because it's a liquid, you can pour it into cuts that can't handle the rubbing friction used when applying the ointment. The oil also works as a wonderful treatment for **inflammation of the nail bed** as long as you rub it in thoroughly and do it on a daily basis. (One night a week won't cut it).

Never, never, never take the oil internally. Some commercially made calendula oil preparations use a combination base composed partly of mineral oil which is not meant for internal usage.

The Tea—While it is not always #1 on herbalist's lists when it comes to internal use, calendula tea does have several good uses. The astringent abilities of the herb make it a good tea to take to help **regulate the menstrual cycle** as well as **curb excessive flooding during the period.** One cup of the tea per day is sufficient. However, if flooding becomes unbearable or lasts for over seven days, see your doctor immediately.

One cup of the tea each day has also been known to **calm an inflamed ulcer** as well as **soothe colitis** attacks. However, for either of these problems, calendula tea acts more as an herbal "mediator" while one seeks a more permanent solution through diet, stress-reduction and lifestyle changes.

Calendula tea works well as a **blood purifier** and **liver cleanser**, straining out built up toxicity. When the liver is not flushing properly, it becomes "stagnant," causing everything from sluggish digestion to a weakened immune system. While calendula tea is not considered a "specific" herb for the liver (that would be dandelion—see page 47 for more information) it acts as a good tonic and general cleanser. Drink 2-3 cups daily for up to three weeks at a time with a week off in between.

Because it works as a blood and liver cleanser, calendula can work for those suffering from **acne** or any skin ailment brought on by a sluggish liver or a stopped up colon. *However,* it is very important to remember that one also needs to seriously look at their diet to make sure they are not antagonizing the situation by filling their body with fatty, oily, processed foods. You can't expect calendula to cleanse or purify any body if you continue to muck up the works!

The only caution is that **PREGNANT WOMEN SHOULD *NOT* DRINK CALENDULA TEA.** External use is okay.

Yeah, they laughed at me as a child when I used calendula instead of the latest brand name. But I held firm.

And I *don't* have the scars to prove it.

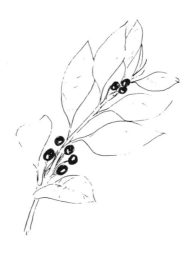

CASCARA SAGRADA— A MOVING EXPERIENCE

Latin name: *Rhamnus purshiana*
Medicinal parts: bark
Forms: tea, capsules

When you gotta go, you gotta go. And when you can't go, life stops.

Constipation.

Just the word conjures unpleasant thoughts. Inevitably, irritability sets in. When it goes on for days, you feel a strange sense of envy for those who are "regular." Turn on the TV and you're bound to hear some poor sap complaining of "irregularity." From out of nowhere, his pal whips out a bottle of the newest, hottest (quickest) laxative and assures him that one dose will "get him smilin' again!" Sure enough, next frame, you see our now "regular" guy bouncing down the steps—tennis racket in hand—announcing to everyone, "It's *great* to be regular! Who's up for another game?!"

Nothing like truth in advertising. Just one problem. For anyone who has had to endure these "irregularity busters" (a.k.a. laxatives), it's safe to say that they only temporarily solve the problem. Sometimes, over continued usage, they can constrict the colon and intestines which might cause further constipation complications. You don't see *that* in the ad, do you?

Ah, if they only knew that there was a better way—a natural way—to break through the bowel barrier. And there is. It's called cascara sagrada.

Cascara sagrada is in the same family as buckthorn bark herb but cascara sagrada is many times milder as a **laxative** and less "griping" in the intestinal tract.

During the 1500's, the American Indians introduced this "bowel bark" to the Spanish explorers who gave it its name. Translated, it means "sacred bark." The California Gold Rush '49ers panned the rivers for riches and praised this herb. They gave it their own name "chitten bark," which when said out loud, sounds like the slang term for what this bark tends to do.

So, why consider cascara sagrada instead of an over-the-counter remedy? For one thing, unlike pre-packaged laxatives, cascara sagrada has the novel ability to actually *tone* **the small intestine and colon and help restore normal bowel functioning**. Regular use of over-the-counter laxatives don't do this. The "toning" takes place as the herb gently stimulates the peristaltic action of the colon and activates its natural ability. Interestingly enough, cascara sagrada has been known to restore a colon and intestine that has been overtaxed with over-the-counter laxatives. Ironically, some laxatives contain a cascara sagrada *extract* but in a small amount. The "active" ingredients however, are chemical synthetics which can irritate more than regulate. If you constantly have problems, see a doctor and/or change your diet to include foods high in fiber which stimulate "regularity." In addition, increase your daily intake of water to flush out your system.

Chronic constipation, however, has been remedied using cascara sagrada in *small doses for two weeks at a time with two weeks off*. A regular dose of cascara sagrada equals one teaspoon combined with 16 oz. of distilled water—a small dose is 1/2 teaspoon combined with 16 oz. of distilled water. Since you use the bark, you'll want to make a "decoction" which means you'll boil the bark in the distilled water for 10 minutes to "squeeze" out the active components. (Turn to page 184 to read more about decoctions).

It's best to take cascara sagrada at bedtime. Also, it's a good idea to wait at least an hour after your last meal before drinking the tea. After that, don't eat *anything* else. I warn you, this tea is not tasty stuff. In fact, it's downright bitter. To cut that bitter taste, you can add a pinch of ginger or peppermint to the blend *after* the tea has boiled. (Adding either herb *during* the boiling process tends to deplete their effectiveness). These herbal additions also can be effective if you feel any minor griping or discomfort when drinking the tea straight.

Cascara sagrada's "moment of truth" happens differently for every person. The average time between taking the tea and seeing some action, is around eight hours. But there are some who say it works pronto while others wait a full 12 hours for results. For this reason, it's always best to take the tea at night so as not to have inconvenient interruptions during the day. Another reason for the nocturnal nod is that cascara sagrada has a mild calming effect which can make some folks drowsy.

Cascara sagrada also works in small doses as a marvelous **liver cleanser and detoxifier**. It has done wonders for people suffering from enlarged livers. It was used in folk medicine to treat **jaundice and hepatitis**. For problems such as this, though, you would want to find an herbal formula that worked specifically for the liver and also included cascara sagrada as one of the ingredients.

Another common ailment that cascara sagrada could be used for might sound strange to some people. However, it does make sense. That ailment is **headaches—particularly dull and throbbing headaches which tend to be worse after eating a meal.** The theory behind this is that when the large intestine and colon become backed up with waste matter, bacteria starts to form in abundance. When waste matter sits almost stationary for over two full days, the bacteria starts to "turn" on the body, creating a toxic condition. That toxicity can rear it's ugly head in many different ways—**low backache, fatigue, joint pain and headaches**, just to name a few. However, headaches are the most common result.

I know someone who started experiencing sudden headaches at work. The headaches got so bad that, by mid-afternoon, she couldn't concentrate. At the same time, her stomach was bloated and she was sometimes going six days without having a bowel movement. Finally, after one month, she visited a local herbalist when she couldn't reach her doctor. The herbalist told her to try two cups of strong cascara sagrada tea before bedtime for one week. After four nights of taking the tea, her intestines and colon finally started to work again and she began flushing out the weeks of debris that had built up inside her digestive tract. By the sixth day, her headaches "magically" disappeared. After that experience, she was a convert and started seeing an herbalist and a nutritionist in hopes of using the holistic approach to treat her *whole* body.

This is not to say that every headache is caused by a clogged colon or that every clogged colon causes a headache. However, there is a connection many times between the two.

You should **never use the fresh bark of cascara sagrada** and it must always be at least two years old. As with any herb that does a job on your colon, you should **never overdo the dose or the length of time taking it (no more than two weeks)** because cramping and diarrhea will make an appearance. Also, **anyone who suffers from ulcers, ulcerative colitis, hemorrhoids or any gastrointestinal problems should consult a doctor before using cascara sagrada.**

The herb is not habit forming (as many other laxatives can be). It is gentle enough that a small dose can **work well for the elderly**—especially those who are confined to bed. However, **don't give it to a child under two years old**—it's much too strong for them.

The other big "don't" has to do with losing weight. While cascara sagrada is in many herbal weight loss formulas, it should **NEVER be used to purge the system as a "quick fix" to lose pounds**. As with any herb, you can abuse them and they will respond quite unkindly. Abuse of cascara sagrada causes vomiting, severe stomach ache, dizziness and headaches. So, please, don't turn one of nature's remedies into a natural disaster.

Many holistic practitioners will tell you that most diseases—if not all—start their life in the colon. That's food for thought. And cascara sagrada could be tea for life.

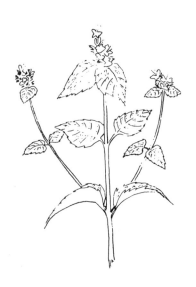

CATNIP—
THE PAWS THAT
REFRESHES

Latin name: *Nepeta cataria*
Medicinal parts: the herb
Forms: tea, tincture

Contrary to public opinion, catnip won't make you frisky. And it *won't* get you high. Give the dried herb to a cat and it's a different story. Catnip can intoxicate a cat, turning a mild-mannered pet into a glassy-eyed demon. Give the herb to a human being—especially a child—and you're likely to get just the *opposite* effect: i.e., a calm, sedate kid.

This fact is important because back in the late 1960's, word got out that catnip was a cheap way to get high. A report published in the *Journal of the American Medical Association* stated that catnip produced "marijuana-like intoxication." They even had a photograph of what they claimed was catnip. Turns out that, upon closer investigation, the reason the tested herb produced "marijuana-like intoxication" was because the herb they used *was* marijuana. Easy to do, I suppose, since the leaves of both plants are similar. However, once published as a "herbal high" in the *Journal,* catnip got a "druggy" reputation which it's still trying to live down.

Catnip must also live down another rumor which is that a tea made from the roots turns the nicest person into "Damien." You can thank the American colonists for this dribble. Apparently, they used to give a strong tea made from the root to the local hangman so he could get in the mood to kill. In all honesty, it probably got rid of his gas pains and even made him a little sleepy.

It's too bad catnip has received such a bad rap because this plant, which harkens from the mint family, is a dandy herb. Catnip (or catmint, as it's sometimes called) has been used for over 2000 years by Europeans as well as American Indians as "the herb" for **childhood colds and colic**. I know several mothers who say catnip tea is the "only thing they use" to get their baby over the colicky blues. Like other herbs in the mint family, catnip soothes the stomach and gently expels gas—and it does so quite rapidly, usually within an hour.

For babies, you'll want to make a *very weak* tea which means *half a teaspoon or less into 10 oz. of warm distilled water.* Let it steep for only a few minutes, then strain immediately. Give the tea to your infant *sparingly*—a "baby-size" teaspoon at a time is plenty to see how the baby is handling the liquid.

If the **colic** has really got a hold of your baby, you can administer the warm tea as an enema. For this, the measurements are one pint of hot water to one ounce of catnip. Pour the hot water over the catnip and let it steep for 10-15 minutes. Strain, cool until the tea is warm to the touch and administer in two ounce increments. The same enema has also worked wonders to **bring down a baby's fever** when nothing else would work. Some mothers from days gone by even placed a small muslin bag filled with catnip herb in the baby's crib so he or she could have the added benefit of breathing in the comforting lemon-minty vapors.

There is also the added benefit of catnip being a **sedative**. While it's clearing up colic, it's also soothing to the nerves and can turn a cranky kid into a sleeping kid. Strange as it sounds, the same chemicals (*nepetalactone isomers*) responsible for making a cat go loopy are almost the same as the natural sedatives that are found in another sedating herb called valerian root (*valepotriates*). Adults as well as kids can use catnip tea as a mild relaxant. It can even take the edge off a nervous headache.

Since catnip does a job on colic (i.e., gas pains), it makes sense that it can also work for any age as a marvelous **digestive aid**. (Some herbalists refer to catnip as "Nature's Alka Seltzer"). A cup of catnip tea (two teaspoons to 8 oz. of hot distilled water) taken after meals helps to **break up gas and avoid bloating**. A cup of catnip tea *before* meals can **stimulate your appetite**. And if you're feeling a little "on edge" because of nerves and it's starting to affect your tummy, a cup of catnip tea can soothe and sedate the stomach lining and take off that "edge."

Next to colic, the second most popular use for catnip is as a **cold and flu** buster. And, like I said, it is considered "a specific" remedy for children. Warm catnip tea has the admirable ability of both alleviating **diarrhea** and helping to **bring down a fever** without further raising the body temperature. It does this by producing a big time sweat which can literally "unlock" the toxins from the body, lower the fever and get you back on track. If the fever is climbing higher and higher and the child is becoming sicker and sicker, many herbalists strongly suggest using a catnip enema immediately. When this is done, the fever will often break within half an hour. This simple process literally saved the lives of many children. Another advantage of using catnip tea and a catnip enema when your child is fighting the flu is that it also helps to curb any restlessness as it lulls the child to sleep.

If **bronchitis** is your bout, catnip could be your saving grace. Europeans have been using it for years to cut the pain of chronic bronchitis. You can drink up to three cups per day. However, if the bronchitis worsens, discontinue use of the tea and see a doctor immediately.

Because of its soothing qualities, catnip tea is also great for **relieving menstrual cramps**. Furthermore, it has traditionally been used to **promote menstruation** when your period is late. Herbs which stimulate menstruation also tend to stimulate the uterine muscles which means that pregnant women should usually not take it. However, if you are pregnant, *with a doctor's permission*, one cup of catnip tea every now and then for headaches or tension might be okay.

There are even studies which show that catnip has **natural antibiotic abilities**. While it is not as powerful as say, garlic (see page 73), catnip can still do the trick. For this reason, you could use the fresh plant as a poultice in a pinch for **minor cuts, garden mishaps and scrapes.** (Mind you, we're only talking about using this poultice until you can get to a sink to wash out the cut and bandage it). To make a quickie catnip poultice from the fresh plant, simply tear off several leaves, crush them and wet them with your saliva. Apply the crushed leaves to your cut, making sure that it stays moist against the skin.

One of the most important things about catnip tea is that you must *NEVER BOIL THE LEAVES*. Boiling the leaves leeches out all the healing oils that are trapped within the plant. So when I say steep, I mean *steep*, i.e., pour very hot (not boiling) water over the leaves and let it set for 10-15 minutes before straining and drinking. Adding a pinch of ginger root to the tea will intensify the action of catnip and act as a catalyst to get it moving more quickly. However, I wouldn't use ginger with infants or children—it might be too stimulating for their tummies.

Call it a lifesaver, call it a gentle giant, heck, call it the "cat's meow"—either way, catnip could very well become a permanent member on your herbal shelf.

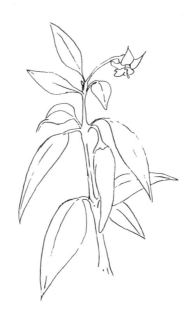

CAYENNE— IT'S NOT JUST FOR BREAKFAST ANYMORE

Latin name: Capsicum frutescens
Medicinal parts: the dried fruit
Forms: dried powder, tea, capsule, oil extraction, ointment, liniment

"That's no herbal medicine, that's a condiment!" a friend retorted when I was extolling the virtues of cayenne. While she was correct in her culinary observation, she was way off when it comes to cayenne's incredible track record on the healing front. In fact, cayenne is so highly regarded, entire herbal books have been devoted to this "hot" herb.

When you think of cayenne, think of "circulation." This potent pepper works its herbal magic by increasing blood flow wherever it is needed. Where there is blood circulating—whether it be to a sore muscle, painful joint or an overall sluggish body—the healing process can begin.

Mind you, when herbalists talk about cayenne in its healing form, they're **not referring to it in its cooked or raw fruit form.** This is important because cayenne in its cooked or raw form can be a major contributor to ulcers as well as a nasty irritant to the digestive tract.

The best and most popular way to use cayenne for herbal help is in its dried, uncooked and usually *powdered* form (although the ointment, liniment and oil are all good). But, a word of caution: when one starts using cayenne powder internally, *always* start with small doses. One-half pinch of the powdered herb in an 8 oz. glass of warm distilled water a day is sufficient, gradually working up to a bigger pinch of the herb. Many people who skip down the herbal path tend to think that "more is better." They reason that "if a little will help me a bit, a lot will help me faster." Try that theory with cayenne and you'll feel enough heat to propel you to the moon and back.

We're talking big time heat. Once, by mistake, I sniffed a few of the powder granules up my nose. It felt like somebody lit a campfire in my nostrils. I tried sniffing ice water up my nose, but nothing worked to kill the intense heat. Fortunately, the heat subsided in 20 minutes, but I gained both insight and respect for cayenne in those long minutes.

Obviously, it is that internal heat-producing phenomenon that makes cayenne such a powerful herb. The active ingredient that puts the kick in cayenne is *capsaicin*. Some chemists have extracted the capsaicin from the cayenne fruit to see if it would be a more powerful antidote. However, the capsaicin alone is often too harsh on the body. Once again, it is the *whole* herb which retains the *whole* power.

And that whole herb in its dried, powdered form exercises a lot of power. One amazing but true first aid use for cayenne is as an *internal remedy* for both **black widow spider bites** and **bee stings**. The special concoction is made by placing one teaspoon of cayenne powder in 5 oz. of warm water, then adding a teaspoon each of apple cider vinegar and honey. This should be drunk quickly after being bitten or stung. If you don't have any honey, that's okay, but the cider vinegar is necessary. The formula is *absolutely not* meant to take the place of medical attention. However, there are plenty of stories of people who have used this herbal first aid after being bitten by a black widow or stung by a bee and by the time they got to the emergency room, there were no longer signs or symptoms of the bite/sting. I think it's important to also note that, in the case of a **black widow spider bite**, the formula can still be administered even after one starts to experience stomach cramping and/or the area of the bite becomes numb, swollen and painful.

Perhaps the biggest reason I keep cayenne close at hand is for its ability to **subdue shock** and **stop bleeding on contact**. I know it works because I've used cayenne on many occasions when the kitchen knife danced a tad too close to the fingers. On one occasion, I gashed myself on the palm of my hand with a freshly sharpened knife. The cut wasn't deep but there was plenty of blood. Without missing a beat, I grabbed the dried cayenne powder and poured it over the length of the slice. That probably sounds like adding salt to the wound, but I assure you it did not sting one bit. What it *did* do, though, was short of amazing. Within less than 10 seconds of the red powder hitting the cut, the blood seemed to freeze in mid-air. At one part of the cut, it actually seemed to arc as the blood took on the appearance of molten lava oozing from a volcano and then coming to a halt.

The bleeding stopped but my body was still reacting to what I had done. I wouldn't say I went into shock, but I did start shaking. So, I employed cayenne once again—this time tossing a pinch of the powder under my tongue. And the strangest thing happened. Within minutes, my body stopped shaking and my head cleared. I became absolutely centered and felt I was back in control. The reason for this phenomena is that cayenne goes to work pronto the minute it hits the blood stream. Within seconds of entering the body, cayenne kicks the peripheral circulation into gear, restores the body's equilibrium and centers the body's natural reactions brought on by shock. Cayenne may not be a cure-all for serious shock brought on by sudden accidents. However, it can definitely take the edge off mental anguish and allow you to focus.

The partnership between cayenne and blood is a strong and fruitful one. In fact, think of most any ailment that has to do with **blood flow and/or circulation** and cayenne might be able to help.

For example, cayenne has the ability to prevent internal **blood clots**. Researchers sparked onto this idea when they discovered that residents of Thailand hardly have any blood clotting problems. The reason: their higher than normal consumption of cayenne-laced food. The dose is one cayenne capsule a day *with meals*, working up to two capsules a day as maintenance.

Varicose veins are often the result of poor blood circulation and even clotting concerns. Cayenne might just help on this front, too. A pinch of the powder mixed in hot distilled water or juice and taken first thing in the morning is the recommended dose. You can work up to taking this concoction twice a day (morning and early afternoon) after about two weeks. If the taste is disagreeable, feel free to stir in a half pinch of ginger root powder. This will take the edge off the taste and also add a burst of circulating power.

Since the heart is the main organ for circulating blood throughout the body, cayenne can be a great asset. In fact, there are those who feel cayenne's ability to help **tone and strengthen the heart** is nothing short of amazing. Mind you, if you have a serious heart condition, medical attention should always be your first course of action. However, a daily pinch of powdered cayenne in a glass of hot water or tomato juice (preferably taken first thing in the morning on an empty stomach) will act as an overall tonic, increasing stamina while supporting the heart.

Believe it or not, this incredible herb has also been responsible for saving the lives of people who suffered a **heart attack**. There have been cases where someone having a heart attack was quickly administered pinches of powdered cayenne directly on their tongue. Within a matter of seconds, the pain subsided. No, cayenne is not the "cure" for a heart attack. Rather, it can help bring a victim back from the brink while they await medical help.

Cayenne has even been found to **lower cholesterol and blood pressure**. It appears that the herb encourages the body to excrete cholesterol and fat. The lower your fat count, the more likely your blood pressure will be reduced. One can either take a capsule of cayenne powder during a high-fat meal or—better yet—dissolve one or two pinches of powdered cayenne in an 8 oz. glass of tomato juice and drink up!

This mighty powdered pepper can also quickly **reduce blood sugar levels**. Instead of the usual lab rat, a pack of dogs were picked off the streets in Kingston, Jamaica and given powdered cayenne herb. Almost immediately, according to the study, the poochs' blood sugar dropped and stayed that way for several hours. The theory behind this is that **diabetics** can benefit from an average of three cayenne capsules a day. As with any chronic ailment, such as diabetes, I strongly suggest you consult your doctor before packin' that powder into your daily routine.

There are lots of other things this herb can do—some of which have the "blood connection" and some of which have the "cayenne heat" connection.

Ulcers, strangely enough, have been helped by cayenne. As I mentioned before, the cooked or raw fruit form is a no-no for ulcer sufferers. However, that powder can do the trick. It might sound like adding kindling to the fire to suggest cayenne for ulcer treatment. But one cayenne capsule or a pinch of the powdered herb in 8 oz. of warm water, taken twice a day *during* meals has been found to stimulate the stomach's mucosal cells which, in turn, produces loads of mucus. The mucus coats the walls of the intestines and flows over those angry ulcers. Because cayenne coats, it soothes. However, without a change in diet, attitude and stress-reduction, the ulcers will remain.

Old folk remedies tout cayenne as the one herb that can knock out a cold faster than white lightning. Many **cold and flu** recipes include chicken soup with several garlic cloves and a "pinch of cayenne pepper." It makes sense, actually, since the garlic works as a natural antibiotic and the cayenne helps to stimulate the body to fight off the infection.

Also on the cold and flu front, if one of your symptoms is a **sore throat**, try gargling with a pinch of cayenne in 8 oz. of water. This may sound like a painful remedy, but it really does work to numb pain as it clears away mucus, increases circulation to the affected area and acts as a natural antiseptic. One idea is to use pineapple juice as the base for the gargle to further loosen trapped mucus. As I mentioned before, when using cayenne for any ailment, *always* start off with a small dose, increasing the dose to your individual comfort level.

They don't call cayenne the "heating herb" for nothing. I've used a light sprinkle of powdered cayenne in my socks during the winter to keep my **feet warm**. Mind you, when I say a sprinkle, I mean just that. Get too much of the powder embedded in the sock and you'll be hot-footing it around town. Another good warmer-upper is to add 2-3 tablespoons of the *finely* powdered herb to the bath water. This heats up the body faster than anything I know. I usually soak in this pepper bath about 25 minutes—long enough for the heat to take over but not so long that I'm wiped out. The only caution here is that if you have sensitive skin, don't soak longer than 10-15 minutes since the pepper can sometimes irritate, burn and blister.

As an extracted oil, ointment or liniment, cayenne herb can be used very effectively—often times, with less chance of irritation. The extracted oil and ointment recipes are found on pages 188 & 190. The cayenne liniment, however, is made by combining an ounce of powdered cayenne in a quart-sized amber bottle filled with vodka. (For a less expensive version, use vinegar instead of vodka). Let it stand in a cool place for 8-10 days, shaking it vigorously twice a day. After 8-10 days, the liniment is ready to use. You can strain out the cayenne powder if you want but it's not necessary. Some people feel if the powder is kept in the bottle, the liniment sort of "eternally" cooks and is potent every time. Store cayenne liniment in the same dark bottle you made it in and keep it on a cool shelf.

The liniment, oil and ointment are all fantastic to have on hand for any kind of **muscle pain, backache, joint discomfort (such as arthritis), sprains or anytime you need a quick dose of "heat."** The effects will last anywhere from 2-6 hours and tend to penetrate deeper and more effectively than chemical, over-the-counter brands.

Cayenne is not without its list of cautions. **Because it has been shown to lower blood sugar levels, hypoglycemics should avoid internal use of the herb.** External use is fine. However, **when used externally—either in a compress, bath, or any sustained exposure—be careful to not overdo since blistering can occur. Fair or sensitive-skinned folks should take care when using cayenne externally in** *any* **form since that type of skin tends to react much more quickly to cayenne's heating action.**

Avoid cayenne during pregnancy as well as while breast-feeding. Culinary amounts are even not recommended. Excessive doses of cayenne (more than five capsules per day for months at a time) have caused gastroenteritis and liver damage. **I'm also not a big fan of taking cayenne in capsule form**

since the capsules have a tendency to break open way before they reach the stomach. For anyone who has experienced this painful process, you know full well you never want to go through it again. If you do experience burning or pain in your stomach after taking cayenne in any form, the quickest antidote is several swallows of milk or a few bites of any milk product such as yogurt or cottage cheese. If these aren't available, a cup of hot chamomile tea, sipped slowly, can do the trick.

To paraphrase an old slogan, when it comes to cayenne, "A little dot'll do ya!"

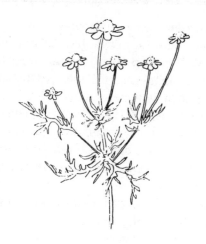

I'D WALK A MILE FOR SOME CHAMOMILE

Latin name: *Matricaria chamomilla (German)*
Anthemis nobilis (Roman)
Medicinal parts: flowers
Forms: tea, oil extraction, ointment, pure essential oil

Even if one doesn't know diddly about herbs, chances are everyone has heard about chamomile. We've all seen the little chamomile tea box at the market with puffy white clouds floating around the lid. But, trust me, this wisp of a flower can do so much more than put you to sleep.

The ancient Egyptians really thought highly of chamomile because barrels of the stuff were found stored in back rooms. Someone must have tipped off the Germans, too, because they consider chamomile "alles zutraut" ("capable of anything"). And those dashing Vikings! When they weren't pillaging, they were soaking their blond locks in chamomile tea to add luster, shine and manageability.

There are two varieties of chamomile: German and Roman. Both are very effective, however the German variety is considered to be more potent and superior. You can use the herb in five forms: tea, extracted oil, ointment, pure essential oil and homeopathic tablets. First, we'll start with the tea.

The most popular use for chamomile is as a **gentle sleep aid**. It **soothes jangled nerves**, **lessens anxiety** and **helps subdue irritability and even anger**. The important thing to remember when making chamomile tea is **DO NOT BOIL THE FLOWERS!** Hidden within each tiny flower is a volatile oil which helps chamomile do its stuff. When you boil chamomile flowers (or *any* flowers for that matter), you leech the healing oil out of the plant, causing the plant to lose much of its potency. So, make an infusion, (with the standard one teaspoon of tea to 8 oz. of hot distilled water) steep it for 10 minutes, strain and enjoy. If you're using chamomile tea bags, stick two bags into the water, set them aside until cool and then place them over your eyes while you rest.

If you really want to go whole hog, drink the tea, do the tea bag eye treatment *and* take a chamomile bath. To make the bath, heat up three to four quarts of tap water until almost boiling. Turn off the burner and add one cup of chamomile flowers. Steep for 20 minutes, covered. Strain and add to a hot bath. The aroma—slightly apple-like—may be all a person needs to feel calm and drift off to sleep. Kids really respond to chamomile and its effects. 1. Take one child, filled with anger/anxiety/worry/restlessness. 2. Deposit child in chamomile bath. 3. You may see a calmer kid emerge.

Feel free to give the child a cup of chamomile tea in addition to the bath if they are really on the tear. However, you will want to gauge the amount of tea to water ratio according to their weight. To learn how to do this, check out page 162 and question #6 under "Clark's Rule." Most kids don't mind the taste of chamomile tea. However, for those little ones who hand the cup back to you with a twisted expression on their face, add equal parts apple juice to the tea. Often times, the sweetness of the apple juice will cut the taste of the chamomile. The only time this could backfire in regards to calming down the child would be if the apple juice was loaded with artificial sugar—so try to use a natural apple juice blend.

Another well-known use for chamomile is as a **digestive aid**. Along with **improving appetite**, this herb helps out whenever **gas pains** arise, **especially when they are centered around the navel**. Chamomile also works as a **gentle laxative**, without the purging feeling.

Speaking of gas, how about **colic**? Many mothers have relied on a chamomile fomentation to quiet their child's colic pains.

(Follow the directions for making a fomentation on page 187). It's a good idea to place a dry towel over the fomentation to keep the heat locked in. Repeat when the fomentation cools down.

As long as we're in the stomach area, chamomile can also be a tremendous aid if you're suffering from **gastritis, upset/nervous stomach** and even **ulcers** because of its legendary **anti-inflammatory abilities**. Of course, each of these ailments stems from considerable anxiety and chamomile alone can't erase the problem. Addressing the anxiety and working it out can.

Chamomile is probably one of *the* most recognized herbs for "women's complaints." (The old herb manuals loved to lump such ailments into the "hysteria" category). The Latin name for German chamomile, *Matricaria chamomilla,* is rooted in the word "mater" which means "mother." Some herb books personalize chamomile by saying that it **works well for women who fit the "touchy, over-sensitive and timid" profile**. Drinking **HOT** chamomile tea during menstruation can help **alleviate cramping and relax tight muscles**. Drinking **COLD** chamomile tea tends to **promote menstruation**. Used regularly (i.e. one to two cups a day) the tea has been known to **regulate periods**. However, if a woman is taking prescription medication either for "female problems" or other ailments, this could inhibit the tea's effectiveness.

Cystitis, another fun-filled malady, can be helped by drinking four to five cups of chamomile tea a day for no longer than three days. If there is no improvement after three days, go to your doctor. Word of caution here: drinking large amounts of chamomile tea—either hot or cold—can cause vomiting. So, don't overdo a good thing, okay?

One of the more unusual yet often effective uses for chamomile tea (in its tea bag form) is as **an eye pack for relief of irritating sties**. A sty is an inflamed swelling—often looking like a pimple—which grows on the rim of the eyelid. Some doctors feel it comes from eye strain while others think it comes from some sort of irritation to the eye lid. Some holistic practitioners feel sties are the result of a sluggish bloodstream. Whatever the cause may be, gently placing a warm chamomile tea bag over the sty for 10-20 minutes has helped to reduce the swelling. However, in some cases, the chamomile tea bag works more as a "pulling" compress, quickly bringing the sty to a head. If the sty does come to a head, DO NOT

PRESS IT TO RELEASE THE CONGESTION. Rather, let nature work its course until the sty is gone. If the "pimple" naturally bursts, it can be very helpful to irrigate your eye with a saline solution. Generally, sties take some time to completely clear. The chamomile tea bag can simply help speed the process.

The tea has a surprising effect for people who have used antibiotics and drugs (legal and otherwise) over a long period of time and are trying to cleanse their body. Chamomile helps to **kill certain bacterial toxins while calming the spirit**. In addition, blending lactose (milk sugar) in the tea rebuilds the intestinal flora that drugs and antibiotics tend to suck out of the system.

Used in a steam inhalation, dried or fresh chamomile flowers work to clear up **sinus infections, head congestion** and **acne**. Combine a handful of chamomile flowers in a bowl of very hot water. Drape a towel over your head and deeply breathe in the vapors. Try to spend at least 15 to 20 minutes under the towel, taking short breaks of cool air. For sinus congestion or infection, you can do this up to three times a day, using a fresh batch of chamomile flowers each time.

Chamomile oil extraction is made from the flowers of the plant. (See page 190 on how to make it yourself). It works as a great massage or rubbing oil for **sprains, painful joints, calluses and swollen wrists, elbows and ankles**. An added benefit is that the sweet aroma has a calming effect on many people.

The cheery light yellow ointment is a gentle but effective remedy for **insect bites, surface scrapes, cuts and itching eczema**. It is often difficult to find pure chamomile ointment that doesn't have a bevy of other herbs or chemical preservatives mixed with it. For this reason, you might want to prepare a homemade batch. (See page 188 for directions).

Chamomile pure essential oil is wonderful to use. There are two kinds of chamomile pure essential oil: German chamomile (sometimes also referred to as "Blue" or "Moroccan") which takes on an intense cobalt blue color and Roman chamomile which has a lighter blue color. Unfortunately, chamomile essential oil can be quite pricey. One half ounce of the pure stuff goes for $40.00-$60.00! Fortunately, it only takes 1-4 drops for the essential oil to activate.

Different herbalists will have varying opinions on whether the German variety is better than the Roman or vice versa. Both aid in calming and soothing both the spirit as well as the skin. Both also have a potent compound called *azulene* which is considered to be the active healing principle in the oil. Interestingly, *azulene*—which when isolated and examined looks like deep blue crystals—is only formed when the flower has been carefully steam distilled to create the essential oil. (Trace amounts of *azulene* have also been found in the dried chamomile flower). *Azulene* is more present in German chamomile, which accounts for its deeper blue color. Thus, many herbalists and aromatherapists feel that German chamomile has greater healing potential. Personally, I prefer German chamomile simply because it takes less of it to create the desired healing effect. An interesting side note is that in Germany, where herbal medicine is practiced right alongside "traditional" medicine, chamomile essential oil comes in varying potencies. "Potencies" refer here to the degree of calming and soothing one requires. Since German essential oils can be taken internally—unlike American-processed essential oils which should *never* be used internally—medical professionals suggest specific chamomile oil potencies depending upon the ailment being treated. Ailments where chamomile essential oil might be prescribed for internal use include high blood pressure and hypertension.

The oil's active ingredient, *azulene*, has been researched and found to possess medically-proven **anti-inflammatory properties** that can **relieve muscle pain, joint pain and backache pain** that would fall into the category of **feeling "dull" rather than "sharp."** In addition, *azulene* also aids in reducing the pain and healing **minor burns**. Just like the tea, both chamomile essential oils also work on the **nervous system**, relaxing tense muscles. **Migraine** sufferers might find a bit of relief by rubbing four drops of the oil on their forehead and the back of their neck.

Kids seem to respond emotionally to the oil as much as the tea when it comes to calming them. One or two drops on a toddler's tummy has been known to quiet an upset stomach. A drop on the edge of a youngster's pillow can help quell **restlessness**. Another drop on their shirt collar can take the edge off a nervous child without making the child feel sleepy or dopey. However, realize that the oil's deep blue color will stain material.

The homeopathic form of chamomile is found under the name *chamomilla*. *Chamomilla* in the "3x" potency, is an excellent remedy for **teething** babies. Not only does it help reduce the baby's pain, it also helps to calm restlessness and whining. One or two tablets placed under the baby's tongue usually does the trick.

There are cautions to chamomile. First, **pregnant women should not use the essential oil in any form** since it can stimulate the uterine muscles. Conservative use of the hot (never cold) tea is considered okay during pregnancy. However, I would only drink the hot tea after the first trimester and keep it to one cup every other day. If you have any history of miscarriage or difficult pregnancy, I would suggest against drinking chamomile tea. Secondly, if you have **hay fever problems or are allergic to daisies or ragweed, avoid chamomile** since it's part of the same family. Thirdly, some people develop dermatitis when they come in contact with either the fresh plant or the oils and ointments. If you show signs of this malady after touching the plant, do not use it.

Calm and quieting, yes. But it's also the flower with the power to do plenty for the many.

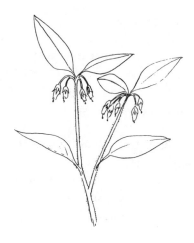

COMFREY—A BONE-IFIED HERBAL HEALER

Latin name: *Symphytum officinale*
Medicinal parts: leaves, root
Forms: tea, fomentation, ointment,
leaf (fresh & dried) & dried root poultice

I sound like one of those annoying "barkers" at a medicine show when I talk about comfrey. "Step up and *feel* the healing power of this *amazing* herb! Watch it pull that wound together! Marvel at how it helps mend broken bones, sprains and tendons! It's *COMFREY!!!*"

But seriously, comfrey *really* is one incredible herb. I've seen outstanding results using comfrey for everything from burns to broken bones. Early American settlers were convinced of comfrey's power and nicknamed the herb "knit bone" and "wound herb"—for its enviable ability to literally draw skin, tissue, tendons and even bones together.

What makes comfrey work? One word: *allantoin.* This "magic" ingredient is an all-natural cell regenerator. The allantoin in comfrey works to multiply healthy cell growth. When used externally, comfrey has been shown to actually "feed" the skin with its nutrients. Some herbalists claim that a comfrey poultice has been shown to penetrate up to 4-6 inches *beneath* the skin.

Taking comfrey tea internally is not without controversy. In the late 1970's, researchers reported that comfrey contains certain levels of saturated *pyrrolizidine alkaloids* (there's a mouthful). Comfrey leaf was given internally to unsuspecting lab rats in *massive doses for two years*. At the end of the experiment, the poor rats had liver damage and liver cancer.

Yet another report in the mid 1980's told of a woman who independently developed severe liver damage after four months of knocking back six comfrey/pepsin digestive capsules each day with a *quart* of comfrey tea. Of course, the red flag went up and the word went out that "long term internal usage of comfrey " was a risky proposition. ("Long term" could be defined as drinking more than one quart of the tea every day for more two months). I *never* recommend anyone take *any* herb in that amount consistently for that long. *The key word here is moderation.*

The main reason you would take comfrey tea internally would be to **break up bronchial congestion, discharge mucus trapped within the lungs or soothe intestinal sores, polyps or ulcerated conditions in the kidneys, stomach or intestines.** You might also want to drink the tea *in tandem* with the use of external comfrey leaf or dried root poultices for **broken bones, sprains, torn tendons, severe wounds or serious burns.** Comfrey is a fantastic herb for all of these problems. In my opinion, to blacklist comfrey and classify it as "evil" internal medicine is unfair.

There have never been reports of liver damage or cancer related to comfrey when it is taken in small doses over a short time. This translates into approximately one teaspoon of the dried leaf or two teaspoons of the fresh leaf (*not the root*—it's too strong!) to 8 oz. of very hot water. Let the tea steep covered for 15 minutes, strain and drink 1-2 cups a day for no longer than 14 days **The only reason you would *not* want to drink comfrey leaf tea is if you have any medical history of either liver damage or liver cancer.**

If that is the case or if you simply do not want to drink comfrey tea, there is always the homeopathic equivalent, *Symphytum* tincture in the "10x" or "30x" potency. The usual homeopathic dose is 5-10 drops of the tincture under the tongue, three times a day on an empty stomach. Continue for no longer than 14 days. *Symphytum* is also available in tablet form in the 30x potency. Follow the label for dose requirements and take for no longer than 14 days.

While comfrey's image may have been tarnished as an internal remedy, there's no stopping the kudos it receives as an *external* treatment. Claims such as "skin growing back" to "broken bones healing in record time" are enthusiastically reported. I might have been a little wary of such claims if I hadn't seen the remarkable results with my own eyes.

There are two ways to use comfrey externally: as a fomentation and as a poultice. A fomentation is made by soaking or simmering the root or the leaves of the plant in hot or cold water and then dipping a cloth (flannel is best) into the liquid, wringing it out and wrapping it around the skin for 10-20 minutes.

A comfrey poultice can be made either from the fresh, fuzzy leaves or the dried, powdered root. A comfrey leaf poultice is made by tearing off one to two comfrey leaves, adding a dash of cold water and gently crushing the leaves between your hands to release the plant's juice. The leaves are then wrapped around the affected part of the body and held in place for 1-2 hours.

A comfrey root poultice is made by combining 2-3 tablespoons of the *dried, powdered root* with just enough boiling water to form a thick paste. A teaspoon of honey is then added to give the poultice extra drawing action. You will now have a thick, sticky glob. Press it between the palms of your hands until it is about 1/4 inch thick and then carefully place it on the area you want to treat. Cover and securely tape with a piece of breathable gauze or plastic wrap. It is best to keep a root poultice on for at least 4-8 hours. For this reason, try preparing and applying a comfrey root poultice in the early evening and sleeping with it all night. In the morning, it might be hard as a rock and that's just fine. Toss it in the trash and reapply once again that evening if necessary. Never re-use an old poultice.

So when does one get to use comfrey in all its external glory? Here are five of the top ailments (and five reasons to keep comfrey close at hand.)

Sprains—You can either use the fomentation, fresh leaf poultice or root poultice for sprains. However, the dried root poultice, which contains jumbo amounts of the active healing ingredient allantoin, is your best bet. A friend of mine sprained her ankle during aerobics class. Within two hours, her foot was swelling up faster than a mosquito in July. Her doctor examined the foot and found no broken bones but a "significant sprain with pulled tendons" He told her to expect to be on crutches for 4-6 weeks. After she soaked her foot in ice water, she applied a cool comfrey root poultice to her ankle. She kept the root poultice on overnight, iced her foot the following day, kept it elevated and then repeated the root poultice that night. She continued the process religiously for one week and by the 10th day (*not* the fourth or sixth week) she was walking around on the ankle with only minor discomfort.

Broken bones—Yet another friend broke his thumb playing volleyball. His doctor wanted to put the hand in a plaster cast. My friend wanted a removable cast so he could apply comfrey poultices. The doctor thought he was crazy. My friend didn't care. Each night for two weeks, my friend molded a comfrey root poultice to his thumb and kept it on until morning. He also drank one cup of comfrey leaf tea each day for seven days, then switched to the homeopathic *Symphytum 30x* tablets for seven days. Sixteen days after he broke his finger, he visited the doctor again. Suddenly the need for a heavy cast wasn't necessary. My friend smiled.

My own experience with comfrey came during and after I broke my arm at the age of nine. While my arm was in a cast, my mom gave me homeopathic *Symphytum 30x* tablets for the first two weeks. When the plaster cast was removed, and my lifeless, limp arm was exposed, she applied fresh moist comfrey leaf poultices for 30 minutes at a time to the areas where the breaks occurred. Even though the bones had healed, the comfrey leaves helped the skin regenerate and seemed to give me more movement with less pain. What I know for certain is that my broken arm was much stronger after the break than before. They didn't nickname comfrey "knitbone" for nothing.

Burns—Herbalist Dr. John R. Christopher was famous for a lot of herbal things but his "Burn Formula" was a biggie. It's made exactly like the comfrey root poultice, except substitute wheat germ oil for the water. It can also be made by combining three parts fresh, chopped comfrey leaves and flowers in a blender with one part dried lobelia powder. Mix enough honey and wheat germ oil into the herbs to form a paste and then "paint" the sticky goo gently over the burn. Dr. Christopher suggested that this poultice not be removed—especially for severe burns. Many times, part of the poultice will actually dissolve into your skin. To replace the poultice, simply layer another comfrey poultice over the old one. If done consistently over a period of days, weeks or months—depending upon how severe the burn is—healing is often more rapid and the chances for scarring are reduced.

Wounds, skin ulcers & bedsores—Remember, comfrey was once called "wound herb." Herbal books in 1911 tout comfrey ointment as well as the leaf and root poultices as being used daily in a last ditch effort to heal skin ulcers, decaying wounds and bed sores. Some people say that within an hour they'll start feeling a "gripping" sensation where the ointment or poultice is placed. This is the comfrey doing its job, essentially "knitting" together the injured skin as it cleans the dead tissues.

One friend of mine severely cut the tip of her index finger and required 12 stitches. Calling herself a "slow healer," she asked me for some comfrey ointment to "see if it did anything." It certainly did. Because of her slow wound healing history, her doctor felt she should keep her stitches in an extra 10 days. From the day she had her finger stitched, she began gently painting a thick coat of comfrey ointment over the wound. The result? She had her stitches removed a full *two weeks* before she was scheduled.

It is important to remember that because comfrey tends to heal rapidly, *you must make sure the sore is free of dirt or pus which could get trapped and cause an infection.* The older and more serious the wound or sore, the longer the comfrey takes to work. On the average, comfrey ointment and poultices can give relief within one week and can show results within one month.

As far as the ointment goes, I have found that comfrey *leaf* ointment works best—*especially* if it is made from the *fresh* leaves. Fresh comfrey leaf ointment is not always easy to find in health/herb stores so I suggest you find a good patch of fresh comfrey leaves and make your own ointment. You can find out how to do that on page 188.

Hemorrhoids—A comfrey poultice works best when the hemorrhoid is exterior to the anus. Applying a comfrey root poultice—made with hot water only—directly against the hemorrhoid and keeping it there for 8-10 hours overnight has proven effective. To secure the poultice, cover it with breathable gauze and easy-removable surgical tape. (Granted, I know this sounds stranger than fiction, but I have known it to work very quickly. And let's face it, if you have a hemorrhoid that has made its way to the light of day, you'll try anything to get rid of it).

Because comfrey is so valuable, it's one herb that everyone should have in their garden. Even apartment dwellers can find a spot in a pot for comfrey. The best time to pick comfrey leaves to ensure optimum medicinal benefits is either before or after the plant flowers. As for the root, forget about digging up the plant to get to the rich root. Instead, visit a health food/herb store and purchase the dried root. Good dried comfrey root should vary in shades from cream to tan. Dark, black tones are void of the allantoin factor.

As great as comfrey is, it's not going to heal every one, every time. I can only speak from personal experience that when it comes to bones, tendons and wounds, I "leaf" it to comfrey to get to the root of the problem.

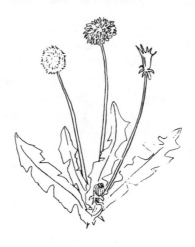

DANDELION—A LIFESAVER FOR YOUR LIVER

Latin name: *Taraxacum officinale*
Medicinal parts: leaves, root
Forms: tea, fresh leaves

Spring brings many things. However, there are two that you can bet the farm on: dandelions and advertisements telling you how to kill dandelions.

I always want to call up those ad folks and tell them that the lowly, common dandelion weed is worthy of so much more affection. While they are fixing up new ways to destroy it, other people are using the fresh and dried plant for many purposes. For example, most folks do not realize that dandelion's fresh milky sap is a fabulous topical treatment for **warts**. With daily repeated use, warts have been known to heal faster than with any chemical preparation.

Even more impressive is this weedy wonder herb's ability to detox the liver and rejuvenate the body. I can just hear those Madison Avenue fellows. "Come on! People don't use this common weed for something as severe as liver problems! Get serious!"

Okay, let's.

Laugh if you wish, but that common, bothersome, yellow-flowered "weed" is actually **one of the best liver and gallbladder tonics and cleansers** around. Dandelion has a high mineral content which some researchers claim **could prevent iron-deficiency anemia**. Dandelion is also laden with lecithin which **may help to protect against cirrhosis of the liver**. Dandelion is also well-known in herbal circles as an amazing **diuretic**. In fact, the slang term for dandelion is "pee in the bed herb." The French, in turn, call it "pis en lit." In any language, dandelion will make you "go" big time.

For this reason, dandelion works wonders to **cleanse your body of unwanted toxins**. And since the liver's function is to sort and sift through the garbage, it gets to know dandelion on a first name basis. In addition, dandelion is rich in potassium. Over-the-counter as well as prescription diuretics often leech the body of potassium as they flush out the system. But not dandelion. Instead, dandelion allows the natural balance of potassium to stay within your body while fortifying your system with this necessary element.

To the taste, dandelion tea is bitter, so feel free to sweeten it with honey—*not* sugar. It's best to make the tea from the root but you can also use the leaves, although the **leaves tend to work more on the kidneys**.

To make the root tea, boil a heaping tablespoon of the dried root in one pint of distilled water for 20 minutes. Strain and serve, adding enough honey to cut the bitter taste. Once again, **the root works on the liver**. You can drink up to two cups a day for up to six weeks with no nasty side effects—except, of course, for that "pis en lit" part.

To make a tea out of the *leaves*—fresh or dried—make an infusion. For this, it's important to pour very hot water (*not* boiling) over the leaves (1 teaspoon dried, 2 teaspoons fresh) and cover, letting it steep for 10 minutes. Sweeten with honey and drink.

I mentioned that you can drink enormous amounts of dandelion tea for a long period of time without side effects. Usually, I always play it safe and keep my medicinal tea drinking to a maximum of three weeks with one week off in between. But the research on dandelion is very clear cut. The only unwelcome "side effect" I can think of would be that you'd clean out your liver or kidneys too quickly and feel wiped out. If this happens, simply cut back on your daily intake of the tea or take a break and see how you feel.

The fresh leaves should be picked in early spring when their mineral content is highest. The best time to harvest dandelion leaves is right after the yellow flowers bloom. At that time, the leaves are softer and more easily digestible. You can also harvest dandelion leaves after the yellow flowers have turned to gentle puffs and blown away, but you'll find the leaf is tougher and harder to chew. Salads are the best way to incorporate dandelion leaves into your diet. However, I suggest mixing the dandelion leaves with regular leaf lettuce and/or spinach leaves since the strong dandelion taste can sometimes make your nose hairs curl. Also, remember to not overload your salad with these abundant greens since they have the same diuretic effect as the tea.

If you wish to pick your dandelion leaves fresh out of the ground, **make sure you are picking them in an area that has not been sprayed with chemical pesticides or poisonous weed killers**. This is obviously *very important* to remember—*especially* the poisonous weed killer part. Even if the area was sprayed months before and the rain has come several times to "wash away" the chemicals, I still wouldn't pick and eat the leaves.

The best way to pick fresh dandelion leaves is either harvesting them out of your own garden or from a neighboring garden (as long as the neighbor has not sprayed chemicals on the lawn). I can almost guarantee that your neighbor will be more than happy to have you snapping up those "nasty weeds."

Dandelion root, ground up and lightly roasted on a cookie sheet on low heat in your oven, makes an old-fashioned **coffee substitute**. You'll have to sweeten this with honey since the bitterness is stronger than espresso. You won't get the same effects as you would with coffee (nervousness, insomnia, etc.) but you will get that "pis en lit" effect if you indulge to any extreme.

A sluggish or "sick" liver can often be responsible for other ailments. Some of those are:

Gout—This is usually associated with poor diet and slow circulation. Gout can be helped by drinking up to three cups of dandelion *root* tea each day. But you cannot expect the tea to do diddly-squat if you keep eating rich foods and consume mass quantities of alcohol and sugar.

The Common Cold—Dandelion root or leaf is high in vitamin C which makes it an excellent tea to drink at the onset of a cold. The diuretic effect also helps to flush out your system. You can drink up to three cups each day.

Weight Loss—Drinking dandelion root or leaf tea alone won't make you shed those pounds, but incorporating it into your weight loss regimen is a natural way to remove unwanted salts and toxins from your body. Drink two to three cups per day.

PMS—A sluggish liver often cannot filter excess estrogen. Thus, estrogen levels build up in the blood stream, causing hormonal imbalances. This physical problem can often result in emotional unrest—i.e, PMS. By allowing the liver to operate at its optimum "sifting" capacity, estrogen can move through without causing unnecessary organ stress.

Skin Tonic—Dandelion root or leaf tea, fresh leaves in salads and dandelion juice (made from the leaves and the stems) is an excellent remedy for anyone suffering from **eczema or acne**. When the skin breaks out with **pimples** or **rashes**, the liver is most likely filled to the brim with so many toxins that it can only unload them through the pores. The results: skin eruptions. Dandelion, in its many forms, taken one to three times per day, may help clear up the problem. Once again, don't forget the diet.

Gallbladder—While I NEVER recommend treating gallstones or gallbladder problems yourself, I can attest to dandelion being a tremendous POST-CARE herb to prevent further problems. In Europe, many people who have had gallbladder problems take what is called a "Cure." This procedure consists of drinking three cups of dandelion root tea *each day,* for six to eight weeks. Six months later, those Europeans repeat the process and many claim it is the one thing that keeps them healthy, happy and herbally fit.

This "Cure" is also done once a year by people who simply want to keep their systems healthy and cleaned out. But the "Cure" is not without some interesting effects to the physical as well as mental well-being of the individual.

The first effect is physical as the body discharges toxic waste through the urine, bowels and skin pores. The second effect is mental. **Many holistic doctors who treat the mind, body** and spirit as one, look on the liver as "the organ of emotion." The theory is that everything from trapped anger to hardened resentment becomes locked within the liver. When a detoxification of the liver is done through a dandelion tea cleanse (or any herbal blend that relates to the liver), **one may experience overwhelming feelings of hostility and bitterness**. Whether you buy the "emotion-connection" or not, pay close attention to any abnormal emotional swings if you do a liver cleanse. You may be surprised by what a cup of tea can bring up.

One word of caution: since dandelion is classified as a "bitter" herb, it could possibly antagonize an inflamed liver. If you suffer from this, do not take dandelion in any form.

What a weed, eh? You may "pis en lit" after sippin' the brew, but you just might say "oui, oui!" to another cup.

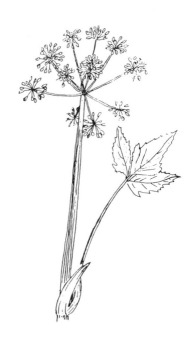

DONG QUAI FOR ME

Latin name: *Angelica sinensis*
Medicinal parts: leaves, root
Forms: tea, extract, capsule

Men have ginseng; women have dong quai.

There's a ton of information about ginseng; there are only bits and pieces written about dong quai. Fortunately though, the Chinese have kept great records on this herb, nicknamed "the female ginseng." From those copious notes and case studies, American women can now reap the benefits.

Strange name for an herb. But since it does have origins in China, I can forgive it. It's spelled "dang gui," "dong gway," "tang kwei" and "tang kuei" and after saying it for awhile you sound like you're ordering an expensive Chinese appetizer.

While ginseng is the male's answer to stamina, endurance and longevity, dong quai is the female's reply to **hormone balancing**. Wow, guys get the stamina-endurance-longevity deal and women get hormone balancing. Okay, it does a few more things than that, but essentially they all encompass hormone balancing.

This is not to say that men cannot take dong quai. Oh yes, both sexes can share in the dong quai magic when it comes to using the herb as a **blood purifier, a brain nourisher, a mild laxative, a gentle sedative for insomnia and a catalyst for lowering blood pressure.** Both men and women who have taken this sweet & smoky tasting herb on a regular to semi-regular basis comment on how, after taking dong quai for only a matter of weeks, they sleep better and feel "sharper" during the day. The latter is due to the herb's ability to vastly improve the blood and increase the circulation. In doing so, more oxygen is sent to the brain which translates consciously into a clearer, less muddled feeling.

But when it comes to those **"female ails,"** dong quai truly goes to town. Some herbalists have even been known to say that dong quai is *the* most important herb a female can ever take. This herb is loaded with Vitamin A, E, B12, folic acid and iron. And instead of floating in and out of the body, the vitamins and minerals accumulate, providing building blocks of support through repeated usage of the herb. This dandy attribute of dong quai will become even more apparent when it comes to menopause (which I'll get to in a moment).

Dong quai is the most frequently used women's herb in the world because it has an uncanny ability to remedy those particularly female concerns: **menstrual problems, PMS** and **menopause.** For many women, dong quai has meant the difference between clear sailing and stormy seas. So, let's get to it.

Menstrual problems—Just as dong quai regulates hormones, it's also a fantastic ally for **regulating menstrual periods.** Many women go through times in their lives when their periods suddenly become irregular. It can be due to stress, changing environments, illness or nutritional deficiencies. Of course, all of these aspects should be considered and analyzed before expecting dong quai to "do the trick."

I've found the best way to use dong quai as a menstrual regulator is to start taking it on the first day of ovulation. The normal dose is 20 drops of the extract under the tongue or diluted in distilled water, taken first thing in the morning. Continue with this simple program until your period starts—which should usually be 14-16 days after the first day of ovulation. However, if your period starts earlier or later than that after taking the herb, chalk it up to the dong quai phenomenon.

Dong quai has a kind of inner clock within its little root which taps into your individual body clock. Because of this unusual ability, the herb tends to start the menstrual cycle based upon what signals your body is communicating to it. For this reason, you may start taking dong quai upon ovulation and start your period 10 days later. Or perhaps the opposite would be true and your period might start a full 18 days later. If you repeat the process for several months (taking the herb upon ovulation and continuing until the beginning of your period), you will gradually notice how your body adapts itself to a regular cycle. Often times, it takes only one or two months for the body to become regulated.

Another added benefit of taking dong quai extract from ovulation until the beginning of the period is that it tends to **reduce and even eliminate bloating, leg cramping and overall body aches**. I know many people who, after using the extract as mentioned, literally sail through their periods without a twinge of discomfort.

If your period starts just fine but pain and bloating is your malady, the above "ovulation to period" dose can really help. However, if you are reading this while suffering through period pain, one cup of dong quai tea (1/2 teaspoon to 8 oz. of distilled water) or 10-40 drops of the fresh root taken twice a day can **warm your tummy, relieve aches or spasms and reduce backache**.

That same warming ability seems to also show up on the face—**softening the lines, adding moisture to dry areas and encouraging a warm glow of color**. As you are warmed with its minerals and vitamins, it also **eases the uterine muscles and stirs up the kidneys** which can make for frequent trips to the bathroom. As mentioned before, dong quai can be a tremendous ally if you tend to bloat. The caution here is that **if you begin to experience more bloating than normal, STOP taking dong quai since it can sometimes stir up the kidneys too quickly**. Also, **since dong quai has a tendency to thin blood, reduce your intake of dong quai or don't use at all if your menstruation is heavy or if you have a tendency to flood.**

Dong quai can also be used to **bring on menstruation after months or even years of not having a period due to taking birth control pills or hormonal imbalances**. However, chronic missing of periods should definitely be taken care of by your doctor or holistic practitioner.

PMS- Dong quai might just turn out to be your best pal during PMS. Remember that dong quai regulates the hormones and in doing so, balances your body which can, in turn, balance your emotional state of mind. Regular use of dong quai tea or extract (i.e., one cup of tea or 20 drops of the extract taken once a day during the two weeks before your period) has been shown to **decrease PMS bloating as well as any emotional distress**. The warming sensation brought on by the herb works to **relieve pre-menstrual soreness** all over the body. Some herbalists say that chewing on the fresh root can help to **curb both breast soreness and emotional rages**. It might seem weird to chew on a root when you'd rather scream, but there have been cases where this has actually alleviated the emotional roller-coaster, making for a smoother transition into one's cycle.

Menopause—"The Big 'M'". A collective shudder can be heard by both sexes because of the possible emotional ramifications this inevitable part of life can produce. The nice way of referring to it is "The Change." The not so nice term is "The Dry Up." I often get the impression that women are made to feel that menopause is more an unavoidable illness rather than a natural part of life. Doctors and "experts" write books about ways to "fix" menopause with chemicals, as though it were some affliction that needed immediate medication. Listening to all this, it's no wonder that many women tend to approach menopause with a sense of sadness and even fear for the multitude of hormonal and emotional changes that nature has planned. *But it doesn't have to be that way!* By using a natural (meaning non-chemical, non-drug) approach, your slide into "the change" doesn't have to mean your slide into insanity.

Some will argue this next point, but menopause is not simply a result of estrogen deficiency. The hormonal see-saw is what is really at play. While estrogen does decrease and eventually stabilize during menopause, the hormonal change is what triggers imbalances in the liver, fat cells, adrenal glands, pancreas, thyroid and hypothalamus. With Estrogen Replacement Therapy (ERT) or Hormone

Replacement Therapy (HRT), a woman can spend months or even years adjusting the doses to get the balance that works for her. Unfortunately, the body changes on a daily (sometimes hourly) basis during menopause and the risk of dumping too much estrogen or progesterone into your body can add up. It's no secret that excess estrogen can promote (but not cause) breast and ovarian cancer. As always, there is an alternative to the chemical choice. While there is no such thing as "estrogen-rich" herbs, there *are* herbs that encourage estrogen production and help to naturally adjust the production based on each woman's needs.

How, you ask? Herbs contain plant hormones which are called phytosterols. Once inside the body, phytosterols are then converted into hormones. Plants rich in phytosterols (such as dong quai, black cohosh, dandelion, fenugreek, licorice, nettle, red clover, saw palmetto, and even pomegranate seeds) have been shown in the laboratory to act as "hormonal building blocks" which accumulate in the body. The body then picks and chooses the exact amount of hormones it needs to balance the hormonal structure.

The phytosterol elements are so sensitive that they can actually decrease hormones or increase them depending upon what the woman needs at that very moment. Better yet, there have been no increases in breast cancer rates due to the use of phytosterol-rich herbs *except for licorice root*. Interestingly, there is one case where a woman used dong quai to wean herself off her ERT dose and found herself calmer, less emotional, and better able to cope.

Dong quai (as well as the other phytosterol-rich herbs mentioned above) can be a godsend during menopause. Taken independently, dong quai helps to relieve hot flashes. The only caution here is if you normally feel hot all the time, don't use dong quai since it may make you feel even hotter. Dong quai reduces menopausal insomnia, eases menopausal rheumatism, helps to eliminate menopausal heart palpitations and promotes good blood circulation. It nourishes and tones the liver due to the high iron level, relieves constipation and increases vaginal secretions, providing moisture to the vaginal and bladder walls.

Obviously, dong quai is one powerful plant. And as always there are cautions. **DO NOT USE dong quai if you are pregnant—the uterine muscles cannot take it. Another big caution is do not use dong quai if you are prone to** fibroids—unfortunately, the herb tends to exacerbate the condition. As mentioned before, since it is a blood-thinning herb, do not use if you already have thin blood or if you take aspirin or other blood-thinning drugs on a regular basis. Also, don't use it if you have diarrhea. And if you find that after drinking the tea you develop extreme breast tenderness or even soreness, stop using the herb completely. Some women report that when they take dong quai on a regular basis, their breasts tend to increase in size. This fact may or may not be your cup of tea. As always, it's best to consult a doctor or holistic practitioner to find out what herbs your individual body can tolerate during those "female moments."

No, it's not ginseng, but it's one of the most "female" herbs around. And it's man enough to stand the test of time.

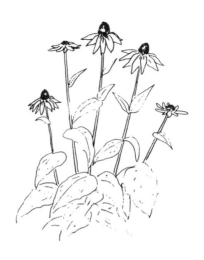

ECHINACEA—THE LYMPHOMANIAC HERB

Latin name: *Echinacea angustifolia*
Medicinal parts: root
Forms: tea, tincture, capsule, extract, ointment, poultice

Rule of Life #153: A good secret doesn't stay a secret for long.

That could be the slogan for echinacea. This wildflower with the tough rubber-like center has had the ability over the years to attract the faithful. Heck, just like goldenseal (a herb which is partnered up with echinacea in mucho formulas), echinacea has a reputation that precedes it. However, like goldenseal, echinacea—which also goes by the names purple coneflower and sampson root—has the "oldest son syndrome," i.e., it's got a lot to live up to.

You can blame the North American Indians for putting the heavy responsibility on this Rocky-Mountain-western-plains herb. It was "the healing root" for many tribes, able to mend infected wounds, cleanse the blood and crack a fever faster than the medicine man could say a prayer. Tribes, including the Sioux, even used it to treat snake bites by packing the bite with the fresh scraped root.

It didn't take those frontier folks long to catch onto this herb. Pretty soon, it was grown in gardens from Kansas to Colorado, made into teas and tinctures and considered as common in every household as an aspirin bottle is today. Even the Europeans— especially the Germans—fell head over heals for echinacea. But 'round about 1920, when "modern medicine" sashayed into the forefront, echinacea was put down as a worthless root. It was forgotten until the early 1970's when herbs started making a big comeback in society. Test upon test was done on specific herbs to try to scientifically validate their usefulness. Echinacea didn't just pass the tests—it exceeded many scientist's dreams.

This plant has amazing abilities—the most important of which is the ability to **boost the immune system**. In a nutshell, echinacea literally forms an almost impenetrable shield against invading germs before they can poke their mangy heads into the body's tissue. Scientists discovered that echinacea actually releases it's own virus-fighting chemicals which increase the production of T-cells (those infection fighting fellows) and protect the white cells up to 30% more than other immune-boosting drugs. In plain talk, echinacea is like having a big, burly bodyguard who doesn't let anyone hurt you.

So you say, "Hey, I'll take this stuff every darn day of my life and I'll never get sick. *Ever!*" Well, many people from Munich to Milwaukee are "daily dosers" of echinacea—shooting a couple squirts of the tincture into a glass of water every morning and drinking it down on an empty stomach. And yes, many folks who do it don't get sick as often. However, new research has shown that constantly filling your body with this heavyweight herb may not be your best defense against ills and chills. In fact, *research has found that after 14 consecutive days of taking echinacea, the herb loses effectiveness.* Your body becomes saturated with it and when you really need it to start fighting off the next virus, it doesn't have the same wave of power. For this reason, many herbalists are now recommending that you only take echinacea for 7-14 days with 5-14 days off. As always, listen to your own body—figure out what your individual system needs. When you've had enough, stop. For example, I discovered that my body only needs echinacea for two days when I feel a cold coming on. After that, I allow my body's natural defenses to take over. That's me. That might not be you, so *listen* to yourself.

One rule of thumb that I have found with echinacea is that **it is *most* effective for colds, flu and viruses when it is taken**

the minute you feel the symptoms begin. Often, if you can get echinacea into your blood stream at the first sign of swollen lymph glands, a sore throat or that overall aching feeling, you can bolster your system and wipe out the cold overnight. If you wait one or two days after the cold/flu has got you by the tail, the herb is far less effective.

I mention colds and flu because in addition to being a fabulous **preventative against viruses**, echinacea can really lick a **cold or flu**. Not only does it shorten the duration of your cold symptoms, it also **fortifies your body with a *natural* antibiotic that helps to stop the flu from spreading throughout your body**.

To get the most preventative flu-fighting potential out of echinacea, I take one teaspoon of the tincture at the first sign of cold/flu symptoms. One can take the tincture straight or diluted in 8 oz. of warm water. I then take one teaspoon of the tincture every 3-4 hours. This process usually nips the cold/flu in the bud. However, if your cold/flu symptoms persist, you can continue with the echinacea tincture 3-4 times a day for up to 14 days. Often, by doing this, you can shorten the duration of the illness and/or make the symptoms less acute. There is a powerful medicinal blend which I have used for everything from serious colds and flu to pneumonia. I warn you, though, it's a nasty brew. But it *does* work. To 8 oz. of very hot distilled water, add 1/2 teaspoon echinacea tincture, 1/2 teaspoon oshá tincture and one decent size pinch of cayenne powder. Stir it all together. While the liquid is cooling down, peel the skin off one clove of fresh garlic. Once the brew is able to be drunk without burning your mouth, take a few sips and then chew on the garlic clove. Take another few sips, until you finish the 8 oz. This is mighty brutal but if you do this procedure up to three times a day for four consecutive days, you can protect your body against further infection as well as charge every cell with a tremendous healing boost. If your symptoms include feeling hot, dry and thirsty, I would leave out the garlic since garlic can antagonize the condition. See the chapter on garlic (page 73) for more information.

Echinacea also does a bang-up job on **strep throat and staph infections,** as long as you start taking the herb at the *immediate* onset of the infection. For **strep throat**, you need to be consistent as well as unrelenting with your intake of echinacea. One teaspoon every two to three hours for the first 72 hours is what you'll need to counteract the infection. Don't mess around with strep. If you don't think you can be diligent with the dose, opt for the antibiotic alternative. Strep left unchecked or treated improperly can lead to kidney problems and rheumatic heart problems, not to mention chronic reappearances of the strep infection. To kill the pain as well as the bacterial and viral manifestations, spray undiluted echinacea tincture directly onto your throat. If you want to really boost the spray's effectiveness, add equal parts of licorice root tincture and oshá tincture to the echinacea tincture. Oshá has the admiral ability to both numb the throat as well as loosen trapped mucus. Licorice helps soothe and reduce the inflammation. Don't worry about how many times to spray your throat—you can do it as often as every 30 minutes if you feel the need. Even after the strep infection has cleared, it is always best to continue the throat spray and internal use of echinacea tincture at one teaspoon, twice a day for 10-12 days, to guard against re-infection.

Echinacea additionally **unplugs the lymph glands** like mad and drains out all the crud that's blocking the healing process. Echinacea is, in fact, an A-1 lymphatic cleanser which can unload a tremendous amount of toxins in a very short period of time. This can sometimes be an unpleasant experience especially when too many toxins exit your body too quickly. You might get headaches, muscle aches, joint stiffness, excessive mucus, etc. and that's the last thing you need when you're already feeling sick. So, once again, *listen* to your body. If things start moving too quickly, simply stop taking echinacea and let your body take over for awhile.

Echinacea also works wonders as a **blood cleanser and purifier—especially if a person has had blood poisoning.** Because of its anti-viral capability, it also can be a great help to someone who's fighting **mononucleosis.** And just like those Indians used it, echinacea can also be an excellent **topical aid for cleansing and healing wounds—especially those that have pus or don't seem to want to heal.** In such case, you could use either an extract or an ointment. And yes, the original "snake oil" has been shown to **draw the poison out of a snake bite when used as a poultice and taken internally** but I certainly would only use this as a stop gap effort if I were out in the woods and it was an hour's drive to the nearest hospital.

There has been scientific proof that echinacea works its little tail off to **support and protect white blood cells during radiation therapy for cancer**. It's no big secret that radiation and/or chemotherapy deplete the white blood cell count which can increase the risk for infection. Echinacea has been shown to not only preserve those precious cells but charge up the immune system.

Arthritis is another ailment where echinacea may play a part. The same shield that prevents invasion of germs, also has the ability to lubricate stiff joints and help break down inflammation. This hasn't been proven consistently but it's worth another look.

The root is the most active part of the echinacea plant. It's made into a tea by boiling two teaspoons of root to one cup of distilled water for 15 minutes. Strain and drink up to three cups per day. However, herbalists insist that the tincture is the *only* way to pull the strong anti-viral and anti-bacterial benefits out of echinacea due to the alcohol content. With the tincture, unless otherwise indicated, take one teaspoon up to three times a day in a cup of warm, distilled water and always *between* meals.

The two things you'll notice with both the tea and tincture (actually, the tincture does it more) is that there will be a slight tingling sensation on your tongue and you'll start to salivate a lot. Once, I got hold of a fresh echinacea root which had been dug out of the ground the day before. I figured this was about as potent as it was going to get. So, I scraped off a sliver of the root with my fingernail and rolled it around in my mouth. In less than a minute, I felt a distinct burning sensation right before the tingling started. Then it felt like somebody turned on a hose in the center of my tongue. Even after I spit out the root sliver, the tingling and the saliva continued for a good five minutes.

Personally, I don't care for that salivating part. However, these reactions actually mean that you've got a potent and pure batch of echinacea and you should be proud. But if the tingle gets too much and the saliva starts pouring forth making you feel uncomfortable, you can dilute the herb in more water (if you're taking it in tea form) or lessen the number of tincture or extract drops you add to the water.

Not many people use the herb in its ointment form, but it is definitely worth mentioning. This salve has the ability to halt a **cold sore**, soothe a **blister**, **reduce the inflammation around a wound or sore**. The ointment is most effective when it is made from the fresh flowers and stems. However, this is another ointment which is difficult to locate as a commercial preparation. But if you can find a good fresh crop of echinacea flowers, you can make the ointment in your own kitchen. (For more information on making your own ointments, turn to page 188).

There are also three "no-no's" with echinacea. *No,* **don't give it to a child under two years old,** *no,* **don't take it if one of your cold symptoms includes fatigue** and *no,* **do not take the herb if you suffer from an auto immune disease such as lupus since the herb could antagonize the illness.**

I suppose some secrets need to be shared—especially when the biggest secret of all is that echinacea just might work.

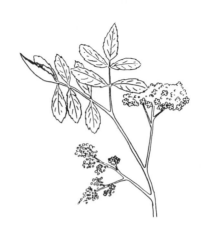

BE KIND TO
YOUR ELDER

Latin name: *Sambucus nigra*
Medicinal parts: entire plant & berries
Forms: tea, tincture, juice, ointment, skin wash

Pretend you lived 100 years ago in some remote mountain holler way past the black timber. You are sick—fever, chills, headache—and the closest doctor is in the next century. Pretty grim, right? Maybe not. Because chances are you'd know exactly what to do. You'd stagger to the porch where the elder flowers have been drying since you picked them last spring. Then, you would grab some of the peppermint leaves you gathered for such an occasion. After crushing the elder flowers and peppermint leaves into a mug, you'd pour hot water over them, steep the herbs 'round about 20 minutes, strain and then drink the tea as hot as you could stand it. You'd start sweating up a storm as you lay in your thatched bed with the goose down mattress and by the next morning, you'd be up and walking around as though you were never sick.

Sound too good to be true? It's not. The elder flower/peppermint leaf combo is one of the **oldest most trusted cold remedies** in the books. The formula is **especially on-target when your fever is hot and dry**. And kids over the age of four can drink the tea, provided they sip up to half a cup slowly.

The elder's legendary healing powers are almost as profound as its "spiritual" powers. The elderberry shrub was thought to have mystical connections and planting one outside your house or barn was a sure way to protect your house from evil as well as bring luck. There is an elderberry tree planted outside Westminster Abbey for this very reason. In fact, there's an elderberry tree on almost every farm in Northern Europe. You dared not cut down an elderberry tree for the wrath of the witches who were said to live in the branches would make your life a living hell. And if all this legend and lore isn't enough, Judas was supposed to have hanged himself from an elderberry tree.

He could have saved his neck the stretch and simply eaten about a bucketful of the fresh berries, seeds and bark because he'd be deader than dirt from poisoning. This is something to certainly take into consideration if you want to partake of the elderberry shrub. **While there are some species of the elderberry which can be used fresh internally, it's always best to stick with the dried herb—especially the dried flowers.**

Dried elder flowers—mixed with equal parts peppermint leaves (1 teaspoon of the combo to 8 oz. of hot water, steeped, strained and sipped as hot as possible) will make you sweat, urinate and stimulate your body to throw off toxins like there's no tomorrow. The typical dose is 2-3 cups all taken within two hours. There are people who use this combo religiously when they get a cold and swear that they feel better faster and are immune longer to another cold—probably due to the amount of toxins the body sweats out. The tea seems to also have a positive effect if one of the additional symptoms of the cold happens to be an **earache**.

Since you will sweat profusely, it's very important to stay in bed and not get a chill. Some folks find they sweat so much they put a rubber pad on the mattress so the sheets will stay dry. I heard a story once about a woman who didn't believe that there was anything to this "toxic thing," as she put it. She was willing to try the remedy, though, and drank her required 2-3 cups of elder/peppermint tea. She went straight to bed and started perspiring so much that she had to change the damp sheets during the night. In the morning, she was over the hurdle and felt better, although weak. When she glanced at the sheets which she had discarded in the night, she couldn't believe what she saw. The sheets were tinged with a yellowish-brown color where she had perspired. The odor was putrid. After that, she believed in that "toxic thing."

The reason it's a good idea to mix the peppermint leaves with the elder flowers is because **elder taken on its own can make you nauseous.** The peppermint soothes the stomach lining and helps the body relax so you can sleep and let your body fight the illness.

This same combo is good for people who suffer from **rheumatism or arthritis—especially if the condition is usually helped by using a diuretic.** The theory is that the "toxic dump" your body goes through allows the joints to lessen their crippling load.

The elder/peppermint combo is also indicated for people who suffer from **upper respiratory congestion and bronchial problems.** The indicated dose for all these ailments would be one-half ounce dried peppermint leaves combined with one-half ounce dried elder flowers steeped in one pint of hot distilled water. The tea should steep for 10-15 minutes. Strain and drink 3-4 cups a day for 1-3 weeks with 10 days off.

Two doctors in Prague, Epstein and Jokel, were thrilled to discover that patients who drank an ounce of elderberry juice daily had better movement and less pain from their **backache, sciatica and neuralgia.** The doctors found that adding 20% of alcohol to the juice (creating technically, elderberry wine) really charged up the formula and sped the healing process. Mind you, if you can't or don't want to drink the prescribed ounce with alcohol, the juice or 10-20 drops of the tincture mixed in water is also effective. Often, simply rubbing the area that hurt with elderberry wine or the tincture brought relief within minutes.

Speaking of the tincture, it's been found that those who suffer from **hay fever** may be able to reduce the wheezing if they take 10-20 drops of the tincture in 8 oz. of hot distilled water every morning. The "secret" here is to start this procedure in early spring (like the first two weeks in March) to prep your body for the official hay fever season six to eight weeks down the road.

A cold infusion of only elder flowers is excellent for lots of stuff. A cold infusion means you pour cold distilled water over the flowers using one teaspoon of dried elder flowers to 8 oz. of water. Use this **cold infusion as an eyewash for conjunctivitis.** Soak a cotton pad in the infusion and lay it over your closed eyes if your eyes are red and inflamed from dirt, dust or smoke. How about when your **eyelid does that twitching dance**? The same cotton-soaked compress can relieve that annoying nuisance.

In fact, elder is considered pretty darn **good for all external skin ailments.** Folks with skin diseases, in general, have found relief soaking the affected body part in a cold elder infusion. Continual external use of a cold elder infusion swabbed on the face daily has helped many folks retain a "softer" complexion. Some even claim it can eventually **soften and "dissolve" freckles.** (No wonder that elder extract has become a prime ingredient in many natural skin products).

The ointment, if mixed in a coconut oil base, has been used to **ease the pain of burns.** A hot poultice of dried elder flowers mixed with equal parts of chamomile flowers makes a good dressing for **stiff joints, inflammation and general muscle soreness.** To make the poultice, take a handful of dried elder flowers and a handful of dried chamomile flowers, place them in a piece of muslin cloth, tie it up and moisten it in very hot water for several minutes. Take it out of the water, and when it is cool enough to touch, place the poultice over the affected area, keeping it covered with a towel to retain the heat.

The cooked berries are rich in vitamins and iron and are often made into jam and, of course, elderberry wine. However, **NEVER EAT THE SEEDS OR THE BERRIES FRESH BECAUSE THEY HAVE PROVED TO BE *VERY* TOXIC.** And since most fresh parts of all the species of elder are considered possibly poisonous, play it safe and **use only the cooked berries and dried flowers internally. Leave the fresh or dried leaves, roots and bark for *external* use if you want to add more punch to your external poultice.** In addition, because elder tends to "purge" the system of toxins at a rather fast clip, **pregnant women should not take the herb internally in any form** since it is way too stimulating to the body.

No, you may not live 100 years ago, deep in a mountain holler with a bevy of dried flowers and roots hanging from the front porch. But I find some comfort in the fact that the same stuff that brought 'em back to life then, can do the same for someone today.

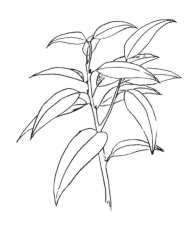

YOU CAN BREATHE WITH EUCALYPTUS!

Latin name: Eucalyptus globulus
Medicinal parts: leaves
Forms: pure essential oil

Think back to when you were a little kid and had a bad cold. Every little bone and muscle in your itty-bitty body ached. You couldn't breathe. You'd lay in bed with your teeny mouth open, sucking all the air you could get into your itsy-bitsy lungs. And you still had trouble breathing. Even though you couldn't spell it, you were miserable.

Then your mom (or "primary caregiver") would rub some nice greasy stuff all over your tiny chest. Suddenly your body cooled down and you felt warm inside. You could breathe again and go back to dreamland.

That greasy stuff was good ol' Vicks VapoRub and Mr. Vicks has made a killing with his product for many moons. Mr. Vicks realized that certain oils, when mixed with a petroleum base, created an opening in the sinus passages which soothed a sore throat and melted away respiratory congestion. Mr. Vicks combined Camphor, Menthol, Petroleum jelly and other "aromatic oils."

Hmmmm. What might be in that "aromatic oil" grouping. Could it be...*Eucalyptus?*

Indeed, it is. Mr. Vicks knew what every grandmother knew. And that was that the oil of the eucalyptus leaf was one of the best (and oldest) remedies for anything that had to do with the **respiratory system**.

Think of eucalyptus first for **sinus congestion, the beginnings of a bad cold, a headache, a sore throat and a fever**. This Australian-based tree which boasts over 300 species, is THE herbal oil to reach for when you cannot breathe.

I say "oil" because you should be cautious of eucalyptus in tea form. Some herbalists will disagree since many recommend eucalyptus tea as a sore throat gargle and a spicy drink to take during a cold. The concern I have with eucalyptus tea as an *internal* remedy is its toxic tendency. One cup is okay. However, there are dozens of other herb teas which are far more beneficial to drink during a cold.

As for eucalyptus oil, NEVER, EVER ingest it straight. It has caused serious health problems and numerous deaths. Some herbalists recommend drinking one or two drops of the essential oil diluted in 8 oz. of water for chest congestion. I don't agree UNLESS the eucalyptus oil is labeled safe to take internally. Most American herbal essential oils are flat-out *not* intended for internal use. To find essential oils which can be taken internally, you will probably have to travel to Europe—specifically Germany—where they distill the oils especially for internal use.

But just because eucalyptus oil is relegated to external use, that doesn't mean it loses any power in the herbal pecking order. As an *external* herbal aid, I cannot praise eucalyptus oil enough! This clear, strong-scented liquid has **incredible anti-viral properties**. Some guy with lots of free time did a study that stated: "Two percent of eucalyptus oil combined with warm water kills **70% of airborne bacteria.**" Translation: "This stuff beats Lysol." I've concocted the above solution by mixing three tablespoons of the pure essential oil with one cup of cool distilled water and pouring it into a clean plastic sprayer. You'll need to spray it around the room at least twice every hour, especially if you're in sick rooms where bacteria is throwing its own private party. Spray it on phone receivers, bedding and pillows. In fact, spraying the water/oil combo on sheets and pillowcases is like a breath of fresh air for someone with sinus congestion. Not only does eucalyptus oil smell better than the chemical equivalents that are available, it doesn't leave any residue and it's 100% pure.

Another way to spray the oil into a sick room is to filter it through a humidifier. You get the combined effect of purifying the room along with the humidifier's ability to unclog the respiratory system. An average size humidifier takes approximately 30-40 drops of the essential oil added to the water. There are only two drawbacks to this: first, since the essential oil is not water soluble, the odors disappear within 10-20 minutes. This means you'll have to keep adding more drops to the humidifier if you want to push the medicinal benefits into the air. Some aromatherapy companies have developed water soluble essential oil combinations which include eucalyptus in their ingredients. This type of oil would be ideal for a humidifier. The second drawback is that some humidifiers specifically state that oils should not be added to the water since they can contribute to clogging of the filter. One way around this is to make a habit of regularly cleaning the humidifier and soaking the filter to clear out any blockages the oil may have caused.

Those same amazing anti-viral abilities work their magic on **sore throats, sinus infection, bronchitis, respiratory ailments and chest congestion**. By deeply breathing in the essential oil mixed in boiling hot water, you can help to loosen trapped phlegm and actually kill germs on contact clear down into your lungs. I've done it. It works. I know it.

To learn how to do a proper steam inhalation, turn to page 192. When it comes to adding the eucalyptus essential oil, *carefully drip 5-8 drops of the oil into the pot.* Anymore than that and you'll get too much stimulation into the sinus cavity and you could become nauseous. Breathe the vapors into your lungs with slow, deep gulps of air. If you have to, open your mouth a little bit to take in and release air. The first few whiffs might be overpowering. Some folks say they have to hold their head high above the pot because the eucalyptus oil vapors nearly knock them over. Try to stay with it for at least 10 minutes (although 20 minutes is best). If you need to take a break, cover the pot since the volatile oils evaporate very quickly in the hot water. As the minutes pass, the sharp odor will soon dissipate and it will be easier to take.

Afterward, if you're still feeling feverish, soak a washcloth in cool water, sprinkle a few drops of eucalyptus oil across it and lay the cloth over your forehead. The oil will immediately soak into your skin and you'll feel an instant cooling down. One important point: *do not* bring a fever down too quickly! You can create havoc in the body when that happens.

The only time I have ever had heard of adverse reactions to eucalyptus steams is with people who either have allergies to the eucalyptus plant or who have asthma. **If you have an allergy to eucalyptus, do not attempt the steam inhalation. If you have asthma, test a small amount of the oil in water to see if there is an adverse reaction.**

If you would like to mimic Mr. Vicks—minus the camphor and menthol—by mixing two tablespoons of warm peanut oil or apricot kernel oil with two teaspoons of eucalyptus essential oil. Rub the oil immediately onto your chest and then get into bed, keeping warm under the covers.

Another way to **bring down a fever and soothe aching muscles** is to add 10-15 drops of eucalyptus essential oil to a hot bath. Add the eucalyptus oil right before you get in so the essential oil doesn't evaporate. This treatment, along with the apricot kernel/peanut oil mixture mentioned above, is also a soothing therapy for **arthritis, rheumatism and even measles**. For measles, you may need to repeat the eucalyptus bath and oil mixture up to three times a day to see some real results. Besides soothing the itching of measles, you also get the bonus of the topical anti-viral properties of the herb which can help to speed recovery.

An interesting **emotional/physical aspect of eucalyptus oil** is that if the oil is inhaled or diffused into a room when someone is feeling healthy, the aroma acts as a stimulant. However, it has the opposite effect on a sick person, becoming more of a relaxant to the nervous system.

One of the best non-respiratory uses for eucalyptus is its ability to keep both mosquitoes, cockroaches and even fleas at bay. For **mosquito relief**, combine one teaspoon eucalyptus oil with one cup of warm water and spread all over exposed skin. To **repel cockroaches**, soak clean flannel in full strength eucalyptus essential oil and lay the material around areas where the critters tend to congregate. For **flea relief** for your pet, take only one drop of eucalyptus essential oil and place it in the palm of your hand. Rub your hands together and then briskly run your fingers through the pet's fur. *Make sure you do not rub it anywhere near your pet's eyes.* While some folks have taken to rubbing eucalyptus essential oil into a pet's collar, I have heard of too many instances where this actually hurt the animal due to a toxic reaction from the oil. However, 2-3 drops maximum of the essential oil placed on the pet's bedding helps to repel those nasty crawling creature. Plus, it makes your pet smell pretty good.

There's nothing like combating one of nature's more pesky problems with another part of nature—namely, an herb. Your pet will thank you. And he or she might also get rid of that annoying wheeze, too.

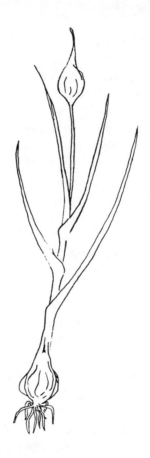

Gads! It's Garlic!

Latin name: *Allium sativum*
Medicinal parts: the bulb
Forms: raw bulb, capsule, extracted oil

When I told a friend that a clove or two of fresh garlic each day could build an invisible shield against galloping germs, she considered the idea. Then she said, "That makes sense. Because everybody—sick or not sick—won't want to get near you!"

Good point.

Still, I can't say enough about this ***natural* antibiotic.** That's right: antibiotic. But unlike chemical antibiotics, garlic won't rob your system of vital nutrients and vitamins. I'm not saying pharmaceutical antibiotics don't have a place in the healing world—

there are times when you need a strong drug to knock out an infection. But relying on them continually for the slightest cold or flu symptoms will strip the body of it's ability to fight the next invading germ. Before you know it, your system is left raw and unprotected.

Garlic works differently on the body—both as a **preventative and a healing helper when the flu bug bites.** Don't take my word for it—take a look at history. During the plague of 1772 which ravaged the population in Marseilles, four thieves roamed the streets, plundering the infected, dead bodies for riches. Never once did they contract the deadly virus. When they were arrested, the officials wanted to know what "magic" potion they used to fight the plague. They confessed the magic was a simple combo of fresh garlic cloves marinated in wine vinegar.

Garlic made heroic appearances throughout both World Wars when the availability of antibiotics was scarce. Fresh garlic was cut and pressed onto wounds to disinfect them and prevent gangrene. The Soviet army thought so highly of garlic they nicknamed it "Russian penicillin."

What's the zip that adds the zing to this beloved bulb? It's called "allicin." Allicin is what gives garlic that sharp, blistering burn when you bite into a fresh clove. It is, in fact, activated *only* when the clove is broken by a knife or your teeth. Allicin is actually garlic's own defense system against invading bacteria, mold and even insects. When bugs try to burrow into the bulb, the clove is pierced, the allicin is released and the bug meets its Maker.

What allicin does for humans is quite the opposite. Besides **strengthening the immune system, garlic helps lower high blood pressure, lower cholesterol, attack sinus infections and aid in the fight of most internal and external infections**. One Romanian study found that high doses of garlic have been able to **detoxify lead and heavy metal poisoning** from some people.

But you're saying "It stinks!" And I say, eat a clove or two, chew on parsley and then drink a cup of cardamon tea. Both the parsley and the tea help to dissipate garlic's after-effect. Forget about the "odorless" garlic capsules. They are worthless when it comes to generating any antibiotic abilities. **Only the *fresh clove* retains the highest level of infection-fighting properties**.

Adding fresh garlic to food is a good way to thread it into your diet. However, **cooking garlic—whether you bake, roast, stir-fry or simply heat the stuff—saps all of the infection-fighting potential**. One organic garlic farmer once told me that the minute you cut into the clove, the garlic begins to gradually decrease in its medicinal value. He said that he always uses fresh, uncooked garlic and always within 10 minutes of chopping it up. Personally, I like to press fresh garlic into my food which forces out the juice and helps to add a more flavor-filled punch to whatever I am eating. I've also found that the medicinal benefits are still very much intact using this process.

It's no big secret that it is far easier to prevent an illness than to whip it once you've got it. When I started taking fresh garlic every day, I was able to beat off most of the germs that made their way into my life. **One to three fresh cloves of garlic a day is a good preventative defense when you are exposed to the latest virus or flu bug. However, if you've already got the "bug," you can up the clove count to nine a day in order to kill the infection**. The only "side effect" (if you want to call it that) is that **sometimes when you first start taking fresh garlic cloves on a daily basis, you might experience gas and/or diarrhea**. This can be the body's natural response to the herb and—in the case of diarrhea—its way of clearing out built up debris from the colon. If the gas and/or diarrhea become chronic, simply stop taking the garlic for a few days or try taking it in the capsule form.

I've personally seen *so* many instances where garlic went above and beyond the call of duty. One fellow I know suffered from a **low-grade infection and fever** for five years. Doctors could stabilize the condition but never get rid of it. One day, he decided to try garlic. Once every hour for eight hours, he ate one fresh garlic clove. He encased the clove in honey or plain yogurt because biting into the raw clove will burn the mouth something fierce, causing painful blisters. On the day he did his garlic doses, he stayed off heavy food and drank plenty of water. When he awoke the next morning, he was astounded. For the first time in five years, he had no sign of a fever. In his words, he felt "like a new man." The condition never returned. Needless to say, he's a convert.

Mind you, this story is about one man's experience with garlic and how *his* body was affected positively by taking the herb. Will it work that well for you? That depends greatly on your own body chemistry and your medical history.

When I feel a **cold or flu** coming on, I immediately start downing fresh garlic cloves—about one every hour for up to eight hours. In addition, I cut out all red meat, dairy, wheat products, sugar and acid-encouraging drinks such as coffee and orange juice. My belief is that when your body is trying to squelch a "bug," it doesn't need to be battling heavy food, mucus-producing dairy products, strength-sapping sugars or acid-rich foods or beverages which only serve to antagonize the body's natural healing process. Your body needs a rest. (Of course, that's what it's telling you when it goes into the fighting mode to stave off the illness). In addition to popping fresh garlic cloves, I drink plenty of bottled water, herbal teas that support my body's flushing process, clear soup broth stocked with fresh onions and brown rice and, of course, plenty of minerals and vitamins. Even after the "bug" has been bitten, I tend to take it easy on the above mentioned foods and drinks for 5-7 days. I continue taking garlic—however, only 3-4 fresh cloves per day.

You also benefit more from biting into the garlic clove than from first cutting it with a knife. When your teeth break through the garlic's skin, the allicin is released directly into your mouth and bloodstream, making it a one-stop, flu-fighting shop. As mentioned above, **it's always best to slip the garlic clove into a tablespoon of yogurt or honey to not only alleviate any burning sensations, but to coat the stomach and avoid irritation. To further help neutralize garlic's burning effects, try taking a bite out of an apple before chewing on the garlic clove.**

Another way to ingest garlic is to encase it in a tablespoon of honey. That combo is actually an old remedy for **strep throat, respiratory congestion/infection and even pneumonia**.

If you simply do not want to bite down into the garlic clove, you can press it through a garlic press or slice it up. However, just like an apple turns brown after being cut, **garlic also oxidizes. As it oxidizes, it loses potency with each passing minute. If you are planning on cutting the clove, make sure you** don't let it set out longer than 10 minutes so you can benefit fully from its potent power.

Garlic *oil* is also excellent when used as a topical antibiotic. I've used the oil many times when I've cut myself and needed a **natural antiseptic/antibiotic.** The oil is better than using the fresh, crushed cloves because it doesn't burn or cause external blistering as the fresh clove has been known to do. Mind you, the oil is a little smelly, but it's also fast-working and *very* effective. Because oil capsules are easy to throw in a suitcase or backpack, I am never without them when I travel or go camping.

Garlic oil is also an age-old remedy for **earaches or ear irritations brought on by infection, water, cold air or fungus.** Both young children as well as adults can benefit. Simply prick a capsule of garlic oil and gently drip two to three drops into each ear. (Even if the problem is only in one ear, it's always best to treat both ears so that the infection doesn't transfer to the good ear). After adding the garlic oil, loosely plug the ear with a cotton ball and avoid drafts or cold temperatures. Leave the cotton plug in for up to eight hours. As always, if the ear continues to ache, throb or affect your balance, see a doctor immediately.

While garlic works wonders on your body, it's also a bang up supplement for your **pooch or pussycat.** Adding one to two fresh cloves of garlic to your pet's food each day is a great way to **keep them healthy and worm-free. It also helps to keep fleas, ticks, flies and bugs away from their fur**. The odor, nearly undetectable to humans, is downright disagreeable to bugs and the like. **Ear mites** can also be run out of town by using one to two drops of garlic oil in each of your pet's ears.

Garlic water—made by combining two bulbs of fresh garlic to a gallon of water and letting it sit in the sun for several days—acts as a **natural pesticide for trees, flowers, herb and vegetable gardens.** A light spray of the combo laced across the plants is enough to combat the flying intruders. Too much of the strong scent and your garden will start to smell like a New York bus terminal. Trust me, that's not a good smell.

While garlic is the wonder herb for many, there are three cautions. **Overdoing it by eating six or more fresh cloves every day can lead to stomach cramps and even hypoglycemia (low blood sugar).** If you are already prone to low blood sugar, you can still ingest garlic—just take it in small doses and spaced a couple of days apart. Secondly, **if you are pregnant or nursing, garlic is a no-no since the herb could cause colic in babies**. Finally, garlic is classified as a "hot" herb. What this means is that if you are hot, dry, or excessively thirsty during your cold/flu, do not take garlic since its inherent heat will antagonize those symptoms.

If there ever were a MVH (most valuable herb), garlic would win the prize. Folks may call you crazy for trying it, but when you're flu-free next winter, who's going to be the crazy one?

◊ ◊ ◊

A GARLIC *FOOT* POULTICE ?!?

It might sound awful (and even a tad strange), but a garlic foot poultice is one of *the* oldest remedies for colds and infections of all kinds. History books tell of folk doctors tending to the sick by wrapping their feet in packs of crushed garlic to "drain out" toxic poison. Believe it or not, this age-old cure often did the trick when nothing else worked!

The theory behind the garlic foot poultice is that whatever you lay across the soles of your feet has a good chance of racing into your blood stream. (For more info on this, turn to the foot bath chapter "Putting Your Foot In The Right Concoction," page 154).

To make the foot poultice, you'll need approximately six tablespoons of garlic cloves to cover both feet. Remove the outer skin of each garlic clove. Using a plastic or stainless steel garlic press (remember, NO aluminum!) crush the cloves, making sure to retain as much of the juice as possible. Add six tablespoons of petroleum jelly to the pressed garlic and stir. Petroleum jelly is best because unlike lard or olive oil, it will not absorb into the feet. The jelly helps to "suspend" the garlic and prevent any blistering from the raw garlic.

Saturate both feet with olive oil. This further helps to prevent blistering from the raw garlic. Spread the garlic and petroleum jelly combination 1/4" thick on each foot. Cover each foot with breathable gauze, secure with plastic wrap and put on a pair of old socks.

You *must* keep your feet warm. The garlic foot poultice may be left on for two hours or overnight. When you remove the poultice, discard everything and wash the socks before using them again. (The socks could contain a certain amount of toxic debris released from the pores of the feet).

Even though you've coated your feet with olive oil to prevent possible blistering, it is a good idea to check the poultice every few hours to make sure the skin underneath is not red or burning. If you feel the slightest burn or discomfort, take off the poultice at once and rinse the garlic and oil residue off with warm water.

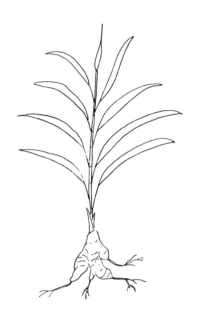

You Don't Have to be Fred to Like Ginger!

Latin name: *Zingiber officinale*
Medicinal parts: the root
Forms: tea, capsule, tincture, pure essential oil,
extracted oil, liniment

Picture this: You've spent a long day pushing yourself to exhaustion. Your muscles are sore, you're wound up tight as a drum and your head is starting to beat "Babba-lu." As you collapse on your bed, you wish there were something you could do to naturally bring you back from the brink.

And wonder of wonders, there is. It's ginger root! It is one herb that has come to my rescue many times.

Ginger root **revs up a sluggish system, warms a body with poor circulation, relieves athletic injuries, reduces acute and chronic pain, unleashes trapped toxins, improves the digestion, helps to break a nasty fever,** soothes a stress headache, calms the perils of motion sickness and nausea and even works its magic on morning sickness. Ginger does all this with none of the side effects that over-the-counter medicines can sometimes bring on.

Of course, as with all herbs, you have to know how to use ginger and, most importantly, how *not* to use it. I say this only because I have first hand knowledge of how *not* to use this herb, which I'll get to in a moment.

First off, ginger is **one of the best herbs for soothing aching muscles and sore joints**. It is also considered an **excellent herb when used externally for spinal pain**. The #1 way to treat the above ailments with this sensational root is to take a hot ginger bath. Consider this bath on days when you've overexerted yourself, feel a cold coming on or need to get your circulation moving on cold winter evenings. (For specifics on making a ginger bath, turn to page 147).

This brings me to the part about how *not* to use ginger. There's a great temptation when taking a ginger bath to treat the powdered root as if it were Calgon. I did this once and lived to regret it. As a former member of the "More-Is-Better Club," one cold winter evening I decided to plop four cups of powdered ginger root into a large pasta pot full of water. After letting the herb roam around in the boiling water for 30 minutes, I strained off the herb and poured the dark yellow tea into the hottest bath water I could humanly stand.

I then proceeded to soak in this ginger nirvana for close to an hour. After 15 minutes, I was perspiring so heavily that the bath water rose another inch. Ten minutes later, I noticed that my heart was beating at a rather high rate of speed. Then a burning sensation took over—not from the hot water, but from the ginger as it sucked every last toxin from my pores. Forty-five minutes into this natural numbness I began to wonder how I was going to get up without passing out. I continued thinking about it for another ten minutes while the bathroom spun in circles. Finally, in a drunken herbal stupor, I peeled myself out of the tub and slid carefully onto the floor where I waited to die.

As comical as this sounds, what I did was stupid and dangerous. **Ginger root is such a powerful stimulant that when used in excess, it can over detoxify your system**

bringing out too much junk too fast. The secret with ginger baths is to keep the water at a comfortable temperature and use only three to five heaping tablespoons maximum—either in the tea mixture or in a muslin bag. Soak no longer than 25 minutes tops. It's also best to keep your ginger bath experiences to two or three times a week so that you don't tax your body too much. In addition, after you get out of the tub, it's a good idea to go straight to bed or wrap up in a warm blanket to avoid any chill to your body.

This same bath is one of the oldest remedies for **colds, fever and flu**. The theory is that the sooner you can rid your body of the poisons (i.e., the toxins that are trapped within your pores) via profuse perspiration, the sooner your body will be able to take over and heal itself. From personal experience, I can attest to the fact that a ginger root bath has nipped many a cold in the bud and helped to bring a fever down literally overnight. It won't work, however, if you get a chill due to the profuse perspiring you will experience. You can easily avoid this by keeping the bathroom warm while in the tub and getting right into a warm bed afterwards.

A hot ginger tea fomentation (see page 187 for how to make a fomentation) works great when you want to **speed circulation to a stiff neck or aching knee or elbow**. Remember to keep the fomentation as hot as possible to generate continuous heat to the area you are treating.

A ginger foot bath—combining 2 oz. of freshly grated or powdered ginger root into a warm foot tub—can be used as often as needed and for any single length of time without risking the "ginger bath effect." The foot bath is a great way to **relieve stress headaches** as well as to **gently warm up the whole body without having to immerse your entire body in the water**.

Another excellent way to use ginger externally is as a liniment. (See page 187 for instructions on how to make a liniment). You can either use the formula which calls for ginger pure essential oil or the dried herb formula. Both formulas are fantastic for any **muscle soreness or stiffness due to physical overexertion or overwork**. The liniment, in fact, is a soothing friend for anyone who **plays sports and finds themselves sidelined due to a pulled muscle or painful joints**. For these folks, consider adding a heaping tablespoon of cayenne powder to the liniment brew. The cayenne "pumps up" ginger's ability to circulate the blood as well as helps generate more heat when applied to the skin.

Internally, ginger essentially has the same effects of cleansing the body and improving circulation. However, it can also be a godsend when it comes to **acute and chronic pain, arthritis, headaches, indigestion, diarrhea, flu, nausea, morning and motion sickness**.

Starting with **acute and chronic pain**, I've got to tell you that I am *very* impressed with ginger's almost unbelievable internal effect. Between the extensive research conducted on the herb and my own personal experience, this is definitely a spice to be reckoned with. Check this out: there have been cases where folks suffering for *years* with debilitating pain have been able to throw away their prescription drugs after one to two months of intensive intake of powdered ginger root capsules. The typical internal suggested capsule dose for acute or chronic pain is anywhere from 500 milligrams to 3000 milligrams each day. It can take from 30 to 60 days to get results, although many people feel a change within the first three days on the herb. As for **arthritis**, ginger's top-notch, internal anti-inflammatory properties make it a lifesaver for those who struggle with sudden flare-ups and crippling pain. The recommended "starter" dose is 500 milligrams a day. See how that works and then increase the dosage to 1000 milligrams if you feel you need it.

Headache pain has also been successfully treated using 2-3 capsules of powdered ginger root taken *at the onset of the condition*. Ginger has proven itself to not only be stronger than the strongest synthetic drugs when it comes to headaches, it also beats the common aspirin since the herb builds up the mucous lining of the stomach instead of irritating it.

A **sluggish digestive tract** can often lead to backache, headache, gas and even kidney pain. Ginger tea quiets any indigestion as it works to break down proteins. If this sounds like one problem you'd like to lick, try one half teaspoon of powdered ginger in a cup of hot water before or after a meal. It could be a sweet answer to a nagging dilemma.

Three cups a day of ginger tea spaced several hours apart has helped many folks get over **diarrhea**. However, if the diarrhea continues for longer than two days, the root of the problem might be more bacterial or viral. If that's the case, the ginger may only temporarily stop the diarrhea or, more likely, do nothing at all for the problem. Remember, always treat the root *not* the symptom. In a case like this, you'd want to try an herb such as echinacea or garlic to attack the bacteria which would, in turn, take care of the diarrhea.

Ginger tea is an excellent brew to take internally when you feel the **onset of cold, fever or flu**. Adding fresh lemon juice and honey after the tea is brewed will enhance it's ability to fight off the initial chills and congestion. Often times, you can get fast results if you also take a ginger bath. Between both treatments, you should be able to sweat just about any nasty flu out of your body.

Just as the tea settles the tummy and helps prevent indigestion, it also has worked wonders for people on the brink of **nausea due to illness or nervous tension**. Some doctors even recommend a cup of ginger tea to patients undergoing chemotherapy to put a halt to the nauseating side-effects.

The same thing goes for **morning sickness.** How many cups you'll need will vary from person to person, however, a half teaspoon in a cup of hot water every couple hours or 3-8 capsules taken every one to two hours will usually help to steady the nausea. **The only caution is that if you have severe intestinal inflammation, such as colitis, ask your doctor first. In those cases, ginger can be too stimulating. I would certainly not overdo the use by taking the herb everyday in large amounts for over one week. As always, consult your doctor to make sure ginger is okay for you to use.**

Motion sickness and vertigo have even been chased away with this mighty fine root. The herb seems to be most effective when 2-4 capsules are taken 30 minutes before commencing on the motion or before instances where you have experienced vertigo. Some people have told me how amazed they are at how fast the ginger works—especially after nothing else "did the trick." If the motion sickness or vertigo creep up after taking the initial dose, feel free to take up to 1-2 capsules every hour until the discomfort subsides. In lieu of capsules, you can also chew on fresh ginger root. The taste can be a tad bitter to some people so start off with a small piece the size of a fingernail. Of course, the same precaution applies—use it sparingly and if you feel any griping in your stomach, stop chewing it.

There is one caution to ginger, although there is some disagreement surrounding it. Chinese doctors regularly prescribe ginger root to bring on a tardy menstrual cycle. However, the amount it takes to do such a thing (roughly 20-28 *grams*) is excessive by comparison to the tiny amount used in herbal tea and capsules. For example, one strong cup of ginger tea contains 250 *milli*grams. An 8 oz. bottle of ginger ale contains around 1,000 *milli*grams. To hit that Chinese dose of 20-28 *grams*, you'd have to consume approximately a gallon of the tea—with the one teaspoon to 8 oz. ratio—and all within a several hour period to get the uterine muscles working. After drinking over a gallon of *any* tea in three hours, chances are something adverse is bound to happen.

Still, the caution remains on the books. To play it safe, **any woman who has a history of miscarriages, should not drink ginger tea. All pregnant women should not indulge in a ginger bath since it can be too stimulating to the body**. A ginger foot bath or fomentation is okay to use.

And finally, speaking of stimulating, **if you have any kind of heart problem, you might want to be very careful if you decide to try a ginger bath**. I've never heard or read about anyone having a serious repercussion from such a bath. However, it stands to reason that if the hot ginger bath speeds up the circulation, thus quickly heating up the body and forcing the heart to suddenly beat faster, there could be some uncomfortable effects. If you have any heart problem and you still want to take the ginger bath, limit your time to 10-15 minutes and make sure the water is not raging hot when you get in.

I can almost guarantee that once you discover this regal root, and learn how to moderate its use, you too will be a believer.

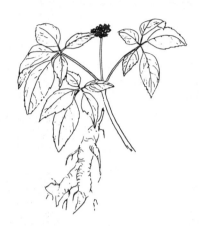

GINSENG MAY PUT THE ZING BACK IN YOUR SPRING!

Latin name: Panax ginseng
(Chinese/Korean/Japanese)
Panax quinquefolius (American)
Eleutherococcus senticosus (Siberian)
Medicinal parts: the root
Forms: tea, capsule, tincture, extract

'Round about 5000 years ago, the Chinese created a whole lot of hoo-hah over a little root they called "jen shen." Soon, "jen shen" became "ginseng" which loosely translates into "the root of man." Quite simply, the ginseng root looks amazingly like a human body, complete with a head, arms and legs. Those darn Chinese boiled the root into a tea and discovered they had greater endurance, a better memory, and felt an overall sense of wellness. Ginseng was a "cure-all" and they considered the root sacred, insisting that the "spirit and life-force of man" was trapped within the lifelike root.

Today, not much has changed. Ginseng still has a glowing reputation that has seen commendations up the yin-yang. It didn't take the health food industry long to jump on the ginseng bandwagon. Products line the shelves in natural food stores that have "ginseng" in their name. They promise "vitality!", "longevity!" and "stimulation!" Some even hint at ginseng's reputed ability to be an aphrodisiac. Looking at these products, one could easily assume that ginseng is indeed the "cure-all" that the Chinese bragged about 5000 years ago.

It would be great if all the ballyhoo were true. But the fact is, ginseng is not for everyone—nor is it a "cure-all". It *can* do tons of great stuff, but there are those who should *not* take it. Ginseng is *not* for people who are already hyped up on a regular basis. While ginseng is classified as a "tonic" and not a "stimulant," the herb can still rev up your engine big time. The difference between an herbal "tonic" and an herbal "stimulant" is that a tonic increases your energy and gently brings you back down. A stimulant speeds you up very quickly and then slams you down very hard. However, if you are someone who lives life at 100 mph and you take ginseng as an overall health tonic, you will crank your internal speedometer up to 200 mph and disturb a lot of people on the road. **Ginseng is usually for people who are weak and/or energy deficient.**

It is also mainly a "man's herb." This is not a universal belief, mind you. In China, they believe that all herbal formulas should contain a balance of yin and yang (female and male) energies. Thus, both men and women take ginseng at some period of their life. For example, in China (as well as in Russia and even in America) ginseng is often given to women for brief periods during menopause to increase their estrogen levels.

However, many herbalists look on ginseng as more of a "yang" herb, meaning it has more hormonal characteristics that fit a male. Since it can work on the hormones, there are those who feel ginseng can dump too much of the "yang" influence into a women if she takes it on a regular basis (i.e., longer than six continuous weeks). If you're a woman and you take ginseng you're not going to wake up with a voice like James Earl Jones and the desire to lift heavy objects. But **continued use can upset the delicate hormonal balance within a woman, causing her to feel "out of whack."** (Never fear! Women have the "female equivalent" of ginseng called dong quai. See page 52). Mind you, I'm not saying that a woman cannot take a specific formula of ginseng on a limited basis as an energy boost, a menopausal elixir or a stress-maintenance or endurance tonic.

There are three types of ginseng: Panax (Chinese/Korean/Japanese), American and Siberian. All have similar properties and all are expensive, ranging in price from $8.00/oz-$20.00/oz. To describe them briefly, let's start with

Panax ginseng—Considered the most prized of the three, panax is specifically **prescribed over the other two when one needs a major boost of "yang" (i.e., "male-dominated") energy**. It is the most "manly" of the three varieties. Researchers have discovered that panax ginseng has elements that almost mirror male sex hormones. **For this reason, women should NOT take panax ginseng.** Panax has also shown a tremendous ability to **strengthen the immune system**. Because of this, Chinese herbalists often prescribe panax to their male patients as a "**fall tonic" to help strengthen the body for winter**. The recommended dose is to take the herb in extract or tea form for one solid month in September or October. Stop taking the herb after that one month of use until January. Then take a "booster shot" of panax in January for two to three weeks maximum. Since it is considered the "strongest" among the three, herbalists suggest two things related to panax: first, **don't take it before you go to bed or you'll never get to sleep. Take it first thing in the morning and keep it under half an ounce so you don't get the "ginseng jitters" all day.** Secondly, **avoid tea, coffee and cola while taking panax** since the caffeine can throw your body for a loop.

American ginseng—American is thought to be **more on the "yin" side (i.e., "Female")**. Chinese herbalists claim it to be **milder and less stimulating**. Often, they prescribe American ginseng specifically for people who **suffer brief periods of acute stress—such as after an emotional upset**. It has also been used to **combat fatigue**.

Siberian ginseng—This is not technically true ginseng. Some herb books even refer to it as *pseudo* ginseng. However, it is a very distant relative to the Oriental and American varieties and gets a nod at the ginseng family gatherings. The active ingredients in Siberian ginseng are called "eleutherosides," hence the name you may find it under: *eleuthero*. Interestingly, **many herbal formulas geared** toward women use Siberian ginseng. If you're a woman and you're set on taking ginseng, consider Siberian over the American or Chinese. Of all the ginseng forms, Siberian ginseng is prescribed the most to help **relieve physical and mental stress**.

Perhaps the most important component all of the ginseng varieties share is their "adaptogen" ability. This means **the herb "adapts" to whatever the body needs to get it back into balance**. For example, if you feel stress, the herb gradually calms. If you are listless, the herb injects a burst of sustained energy. There have literally been thousands of controlled, scientific studies which have shown conclusively that ginseng does do a first-rate job when it comes to **endurance, vitality, and overall wellness**.

Two groups of Russian soldiers were studied using ginseng extract. One group was given the herb while the other was given a placebo. After a period of time, they were asked to run against each other in a 3-kilometer race. The ginseng bunch won over the placebo gang. Another Russian study gave 1,500 automobile factory workers four milligrams of ginseng each day and then gave a placebo to 1,500 others. Over the course of the year, the ginseng group missed fewer days of work due to colds, flu, bronchitis, tonsillitis, sinus infections and stress-related illness. Hmmmm, might there be something in this stuff that deserves a look by Americans?

The list of what all forms of ginseng can do is long and quite impressive. A few of the top selling points are:

- An overall immune system stimulant

- Counteracts physical damage from stress

- Combats fatigue over time as it buffers your body to resist feelings of tiredness

- Can enhance memory and even improve learning

- Has reduced bad cholesterol (LDL) and increased good cholesterol (HDL)

- Aids in strengthening the endocrine glands which helps in the metabolism of vitamins and minerals

- For men, can regulate hormones when used in conjunction with sarsaparilla

- Lowers blood sugar levels due to the ingredient "ginsenin" which has shown to be beneficial for diabetic patients
- Can possibly arrest the growth of cancer cells due to the ingredient "ginsenocide." (This is especially strong in panax ginseng)
- A possible rejuvenating tonic for the elderly, especially those who are not as active as they would like to be
- A possible energizing tonic for vegetarians

Controlled studies so far have only used mice, but the results are promising. In addition, ginseng was shown to increase the lives of stomach cancer patients up to four years. Another plus is that ginseng can minimize cell damage from radiation therapy.

Obviously, this is one grand root. But there are many considerations to take into effect before trying ginseng. **DO NOT TAKE GINSENG if you are suffering from an acute or chronic inflammatory disease. This includes bronchial illnesses and even the common cold and the flu.** Ginseng has been known to sometimes drive the illness deeper. **Pregnant women should stay away from ginseng as well as those with fever, insomnia, asthma, emphysema, high blood pressure, heart problems, blood clotting problems and hay fever.**

And quite obviously, please do not drink coffee or caffeine beverages when taking ginseng in any form. It's like throwing gasoline on a raging forest fire.

The dosage for ginseng is clear and should never be exceeded. That dosage is one cup of the tea each day for one month, *followed by a two month lay off*. It is always best to take ginseng one hour before or after eating. If you are taking any form of vitamin C, herbalists advise waiting a full two hours before or after ingesting ginseng. The reason being that vitamin C has been found to interfere with the full absorption of the herb.

The tea is made by combining 1/2 teaspoon to one teaspoon of the dried herb to 8 oz. of very hot distilled water. If the tea form doesn't suit you, the tincture (5-10 drops in warm water) or the panax extract—which comes in cute little pre-measured glass vials—are easy to take. Overdoses or abuse of ginseng will result in jitters, headaches, skin rashes and insomnia.

Another thing to watch out for is product adulteration. Researchers have found that up to 25% of the ginseng products sold today are "worthless" because they contain either a synthetic derivative or a fraction of the true herb. For this reason, the extract or bulk root is your best bet.

What's the biggest misconception about ginseng? Surprisingly, it's that aphrodisiac thing. A 17th century ginseng user wrote that the herb "frisked the spirits" but didn't produce the "naughty effects." Whether ginseng trips your trigger is entirely up to you. Most researchers say ginseng's aphrodisiac effects are all in the head. Others insist they're located three feet down.

You be the judge.

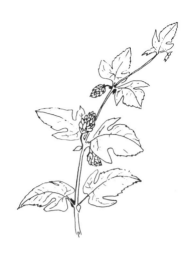

HOPS—THE BEER-LESS BREW TO SNOOZE ON

Latin name: *Humulus lupulus*
Medicinal parts: the fruit
Forms: tea, capsule, tincture, "sleep pillow"

Insomnia is one experience we all share. Young and old, rich and poor, short and tall—everyone, at one time or another, can't get to sleep. Maybe you're nervous about a big day. Maybe you're worried about work/school/a relationship. Maybe you're just so wound up you can't sleep. What most folks do at times like this is struggle to the medicine cabinet and pop some pills that have the words "sleepy," "dozey" or "drowsy" in the name. If those little pills do their stuff—you get to be knocked out for up to 12 unconscious hours. There's just one problem: sleeping pills can get addictive (just ask those "12-steppers" at The Betty Ford Center). And with any consistent use of a sedative drug -whether it is legal or otherwise—it takes more of it each time to get you where you want to be.

If only these legions of insomniacs would heed the advice of the ages and try a hot cup of hops instead. Hops is considered by herbalists to be one of the most **calming and relaxing herbs** known to mankind. Sure, there are other herbs that can get you sleepin', but hops is known to be one of the safest and most effective.

Hops' history dates back to the Roman Empire. But during the reign of Henry VIII—that six-wife pillar of excess—the herb fell on bad times. Henry and his pals deemed the herb "wicked" because it was reputed to "spoil the taste of drink (ale) and endanger the people." Frankly, there is nothing "dangerous" about the herb. Consider King Henry a 16th century lobbyist for the huge ale industry. It wasn't until years later that hops was allowed onto the beverage scene, strictly as a preservative agent for what the Germans called "bier." The rest, of course, is heady history.

However, while all this brew-hah-hah was happening, folk doctors and herbalists alike were paying more attention to the effects of the *non-fermented* brew. Hops farmers noticed that their pickers were dozing off on the job literally. They started putting two and two together. Presto! Word got out that hops was a #1 sleep aid and this beer preservative got a whole new reputation.

The active "dozing" ingredient in hops is called "lupulin" which, along with "humulon," acts as a mild antibiotic. (**The antibiotic properties are stronger in the *fresh* herb, while the sleepy time abilities seem to increase as the *dried* herb ages).** The lupulin gently sedates within 20-40 minutes without any narcotic side effects. For insomnia, try 1-3 cups of the infused herb. The dried herb has the most potency but unfortunately the fluffy white flakes only keep their medicinal punch for 6-8 months—and that's only if the herb is stored in an airtight jar in a cool dark spot.

While this "snowflake" of an herb works on the nervous system, it also relaxes the stomach and bowel. For this reason, **hops is called a "specific" when one is restless due to a nervous stomach or having stomach cramps because of a sudden junk food binge**. Hops can also **relieve gas pains, increase your urine and bile flow *and* stimulate your appetite**. To accomplish the latter, the herb works best in capsule form when two are taken before meals. However, do not take the herb as an appetite stimulant for longer than three days in a row.

But wait, there's more! Hops is considered to be **a soothing pain killer, especially in cases of mild toothache, rheumatism and sciatica—*particularly* when these ailments interfere with getting a restful night's sleep.** To juice up the potency, add a pinch of chamomile. Figure one heaping teaspoon of dried hops and a half teaspoon of chamomile to 8 oz. of hot distilled water. Steep for 10-15 minutes, strain and enjoy.

Hops **curbs hyperactivity, especially in kids**. However, don't forget to also consider diet when you are treating hyperactivity. Things such as white sugar, white flour, soft drinks, chocolate, caffeine and processed foods are definite contributors to the hyper fund. If you want to incorporate hops tea into a child's repertoire, the dose is less than for adults. Mix only 1/2 teaspoon with 8 oz. of hot distilled water and give it to the child a spoonful at a time. **DO NOT** give hops in any form to children under two years old.

Consider hops the "herb of decreasing" since it spends lots of time decreasing (or sedating) actions and desires. For example, **say a person is in shock: a pinch of cayenne under the tongue will snap them out of it very quickly. Then follow it up with a hot cup of hops tea to calm the central nervous system**.

On the "desire" front, **hops has been known to decrease both the taste for booze and sex**. Interestingly enough, a cup or two of hops tea might also **curb the desire for the foamy brew it's known to preserve!** And **if the individual is going through withdrawal and the D.T.'s come on, herbalists recommend blending 10 drops of hops tincture with a few grains of cayenne in a glass of hot water and administering it one teaspoon at a time**.

On the sexual front, hops has been used through the centuries to **restrain "the excessive desires of men when it comes to the female."** Yeah, yeah, it works vice versa, too.

Externally, hops—in tincture form—makes an **excellent topical treatment for skin sores. For inflammation, boils, tumors and old ulcers, apply a poultice**. To make the poultice, take 1-2 handfuls of dried hops flowers and add just enough water until you get a mashy consistency. If you add too much water, the consistency will be too loose to use. If that happens, simply add more hops flowers until you're able to get a firmer blend. Place the hops poultice on the skin and cover with a sterile bandage that allows air to travel through to the sore. Make sure to check the sore every hour. If any sign of infection shows up or you become the least bit apprehensive, don't try to self-medicate any longer. *Go to a doctor immediately!*

As with any herb, you don't want to become dependent upon it. This can be difficult if you're using hops to fight insomnia. If insomnia becomes a habit, you need to analyze what is at the root of the problem. Continual anxiety, fear and chronic worry are three emotional problems that can cause insomnia. Physically, diet has been shown to also contribute to sleepless nights. Try staying away from soft drinks, fruit juice, chocolate and sugar and of course, coffee before going to bed. Hops tea can help alleviate the symptoms of insomnia, but only you can eliminate the source. **Since you should not use hops for prolonged periods of time (i.e., 1-2 cups daily for no longer than three weeks with one week off), there are two ways you can use the herb externally for as long as you like.**

The first way is to make a **"hops pillow."** Don't laugh! Honest Abe Lincoln and King George III slept soundly on hops pillows. You'll need plenty of dried hops flowers and a 24" square piece of muslin cloth. Fold the muslin cloth in half and stitch up the two sides, leaving the top part open. Fill the pouch with 3-6 heaping handfuls of the dried flowers, sprinkle a few drops of vodka or gin on the herb to activate the aroma, then sew up the remaining side. Slip this pouch into your pillowcase so that your head rests directly on top of it. The alcohol releases the volatile oils trapped inside the hops flowers and affects your brain each time you catch a whiff. Some folks swear by this pillow—others say the smell makes them sick. The only way to find out if it works for you is to try it for yourself.

The second external sleep remedy using hops is in the bath. (Check out the chapter on herbal baths on pages 147 & 149 and look under the headings "Tea bath" and "Muslin sack.") Use either the tea bath method or muslin sack in your bath and soak no longer than 30 minutes.

The cautions for hops are few but important. **Because it acts as a sedative, it is not wise to give it to someone who has a natural tendency toward depression. Women with estrogen-dependent breast cancer should stay clear of hops. The reason for this is that German researchers claim to have found chemicals in the herb which are** similar to the female sex hormone estrogen. Not all herbalists agree about this finding and scoff at the fact that hops is suddenly off-limits to a specific group of women who may need what the herb offers. However, until there is more research to confirm or deny what the Germans discovered, err on the side of the caution and use another herb such as chamomile for calming if you have estrogen-dependent breast cancer.

If you're lucky enough to get out and pick the fresh herb, please wear gloves! It seems the pollen residue can cause contact dermatitis in some people. Finally, if you're a "female picker," wearing gloves also protects your skin from the volatile oils which, when absorbed into your pores, can either stop menstruation or bring your period on out of cycle. This odd little "hops effect" was discovered quite by accident when those early female hops pickers not only fell asleep in the field, but also shared strange effects in the "female zone."

Other than those cautions, hops is pretty darn mild compared to those dozey-sleepy-drowsy white pills. You can bank on it and even sleep on it.

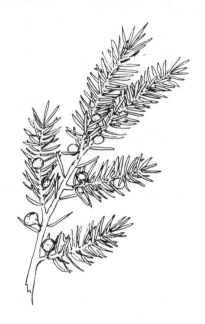

JUNIPER—JUST SAY GO!

Latin name: *Juniperus communis*
Medicinal parts: berries
Forms: tea, pure essential oil

About 400 years ago, a little Dutch pharmacist wanted to make a cheap drink that would help people tinkle. Relying on herbs in his town, he created the perfect concoction. He blended berries from the juniper tree with water and other ingredients. Then he let them ferment and bottled the tonic. He called it "gin" and the public really liked the stuff—unfortunately, though, not for the reasons he invented it. To this day, a gin and tonic will make you tinkle (among other things) and it's all due to those tiny berries that pack a punch.

Juniper berries are **one of *the* best herbal diuretics**. During the journey west, pioneers depended upon these berries to alleviate everything from kidney ailments and edema to urinary tract infections. Today, juniper is used in much the same way. However, it does lots more than "make you go."

First off, **if you have any kind of serious kidney infection or chronic kidney problems, you SHOULD NOT USE JUNIPER. Unfortunately, the herb may only**

complicate matters. However, if you have the occasional bout with water retention or urinary blockages, juniper may be your one way ticket to tinkle heaven. And it *will* make you go, so it's always a good idea to start off with half the dose and work up to a full dose. The usual dosage is 3-5 crushed berries in one cup of boiling water. Let it steep covered for 10-20 minutes, strain and then sip slowly. You can drink 1-2 cups of juniper tea per day. More than that, and you risk overtaxing your kidneys and irritating your urinary passage. And don't be surprised if your urine smells like sweet violets. That's the berries working their magic as they travel through your body.

In addition to working as a diuretic, juniper tea can **reduce edema, soothe burning urination and take the pressure off an enlarged prostate**. It's very important that you check with your doctor before embarking on juniper as part of your therapy if your condition is advanced or chronic. If the herb checks out for you, I would strongly consider combining a pinch of parsley with your daily brew to soften the edge of juniper's diuretic action.

Juniper tea is also considered excellent as **both an internal and external (poultice) remedy for insect bites, snake bites, bee and wasp stings**. Essentially, what the tea does internally is help clear the poisons out of your bloodstream via your urinary tract. Externally, the crushed berry poultice helps to draw out pain and infection. Obviously, if the bite is serious or life-threatening, forget about the juniper berries and get thee to a doctor!

Chewing on the fresh berries will sweeten your breath and has been known to curb the pain of infected gums. Be careful, though, if you go out to pick fresh juniper berries. There are over 70 species of juniper trees with the six to 20 foot *J. communis* species being the standard medicinal plant. There are also lots of pretty bushes filled with lovely little red berries that look similar to juniper. However, take one bite of *those* berries and you end up in the local hospital getting a good ol' stomach pump. So either be dead-on sure it's a juniper bush or, better yet, purchase the herb from an health/herb store.

The berries are also marvelous to keep on hand if you are in charge of someone who is sick. Chewing on 6-10 berries a day or sipping one cup of tea throughout the day may act as a **natural fortifier for your immune system**. In fact, healers from Tibet to Germany used to burn the twigs, leaves and berries of the juniper tree in sick rooms to disinfect the air and clear out "evil spirits."

One can also use juniper in its pure essential oil form. Combined either in a bath, steam inhalation, massage oil or distilled water spray, juniper essential oil can work wonders for a host of complaints. Enjoying a juniper essential oil bath can do a whole lot more than stir your aromatic senses. Taken once a week, **the bath works sort of like an "external diuretic," unlocking water retention and sloughing off trapped toxins**. For this reason, it's a fantastic bath to take if you suffer from **PMS** because it also works to calm and soothe your nerves.

In fact, *anytime* **you experience nervous tension, a juniper bath can help get you centered again. Remember that all pure essential oils work on both an emotional (mental) and physical level. Taking this into consideration, juniper essential oil is especially good for folks who absorb lots of negative emotions from others**. For instance, if you work in a job where you come in contact with an angry public or nervous, frenetic employees, you could benefit greatly with a bi-weekly juniper bath. If it's really bad, you might want to consider carrying around a cotton ball or tissue with a few drops of juniper essential oil sprinkled on it and taking a whiff throughout the day whenever the negativity becomes too much. The bath also works when you're feeling **anxious, full of anxiety or depressed. The aroma can also promote a sense of well-being and inner strength as it stimulates the mind.** In addition, adding juniper essential oil to your bath water helps to improve circulation without causing the over stimulation of say, cayenne. The oil/bath measurement would be 10-15 essential oil drops in a hot tub, poured in *right before* you get in the tub so the vital therapeutic benefits of the oil don't evaporate.

Another great way to use juniper pure essential oil is in a steam inhalation. This age old trick—with approximately 5-8 drops of the oil added to a pasta-size pot of very hot water—works for **respiratory problems and is especially soothing for children with coughs and congestion**. The steam inhalation used twice a week can also help to **dry up acne and clean out**

the toxic debris from the pores. Used as a cheap pick-me-up at-home facial, a juniper steam inhalation can **help to reduce puffiness in the face as well as temporarily dry up an oily complexion.** To top it off, a whiff of juniper (either in the steam inhalation, in the bath or on a cotton ball) can **activate the brain and some say, improve the memory.**

Mixed into a massage oil (for a large portion, add 30-60 drops of the pure essential oil to 6 oz. of sweet almond oil or apricot kernel oil, for smaller portions, add 3-4 drops to one tablespoon of either base oil), the blend can be gently massaged over the abdomen to **relieve painful menstrual cramping.** If you rub it across the throat and chest, the massage oil can **lessen respiratory congestion.** Applied over the lower back, the oil has helped **ease sciatic pain.** Worked into **rheumatic or arthritic joints,** the same oil can aid in **excreting uric acid build up.** Massaged into **cellulite,** juniper can really help smooth and gradually decrease the problem. Add a drop or two of chamomile essential oil to the blend, and you've got an A-1 alternative lotion for **"weeping eczema." NEVER apply the essential oil "neat" (which means right out of the bottle) since it can burn and even blister skin.**

One word of caution about using this juniper oil blend for cellulite. I recommended it to a friend once who wanted a natural oil for diminishing cellulite. She rubbed the juniper blend into her upper thighs and buttocks for several nights in a row. On the fourth day, her period arrived two weeks early. You see, juniper also happens to be **one of the best herbs to help bring on a menstrual cycle.** This example only goes to prove that the pure essential oil really *does* seep through the pores and into the bloodstream! So, beware of the berry if you are trying to regulate your cycle.

For a cheap but **efficient room deodorizer** and fungal killer, in a plastic pump bottle add 30-60 drops of juniper essential oil to 6 oz. of distilled water. Spray freely around rooms that need to be cleared out—especially if someone has been ill.

Because juniper can promote a period, you should NEVER take juniper in either the tea *or* use it in the pure essential oil form if you are pregnant—it's way too stimulating to the uterine walls. Also, one should not take the herb internally for longer than six weeks

without a three week break so your kidneys don't get overtaxed. Since diuretics in general have a tendency to deplete your system of potassium, it's a good idea to replenish your body with potassium-rich foods such as green leafy vegetables, carrots, beans and alfalfa. And if you have a tendency toward hay fever, approach juniper carefully since one-third of hay fever sufferers have an allergic reaction to the herb.

This common evergreen might be the juice for gin, but as an herb, it can do berry much more.

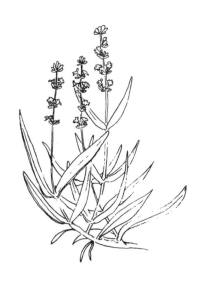

LAVENDER—
IT'S SIESTA TIME!

Latin name: Lavendula officinalis
Medicinal parts: flowers & leaves
Forms: pure essential oil, extracted oil, tea

If you fall down into a field of blossoming lavender, you may not be able to get up. The sedative action could take hold, knocking you into the most relaxed, blissful state. Okay, I may be exaggerating a wee bit, but honest injun, lavender is one herb that everyone should have in the cupboard. And not just for its legendary soothing qualities. This herb—in both its tea and pure essential oil form—can do loads more than send you into dreamland.

It's got a history steeped in lore and legend. Way back in Ancient Greece and Rome, ladies drenched themselves in lavender water to purify their bodies. "Why bother with a pesky bath," they thought, "when I can drown myself in this stuff?" Lavender flowers were picked at the height of their potency (mid-summer when the oil is concentrated in the flower), dried and then burned in houses to keep out evil spirits. Then there was the belief that a sprinkle of lavender water a day maintained chastity in every way. Since lavender is looked on by some herbalists to be an *an*aphrodisiac (i.e., lessens the sexual desire). This may not be so far from the truth. In any case, I certainly wouldn't rely on lavender to dim your desires.

These days, you'll find lavender in everything from sachets to soaps to dried flower arrangements. It is one of the most fragrant flowers and does most of its herbal magic through your sense of smell.

You can take lavender herb internally, although, to me, it's like drinking perfume. The dried herb can be taken alone or mixed with other herbs in formulas that relate to **insomnia, fatigue, depression or nervous exhaustion.** The normal tea to water dose is one heaping teaspoon of dried lavender flowers to 8 oz. of very hot water. Cover and steep for 10 minutes to allow the fragrant volatile oils to release their calming aroma. Strain and drink. As I said, lavender tea is lovely but for some folks, it can be too fragrant. (Two very good non-fragrant calming teas are chamomile and hops, which can be found on pages 35 and 92 respectively).

Personally, I prefer to use lavender for external use. And boy, are there plenty of external uses for dried lavender, lavender pure essential oil and the extracted oil of lavender. (To learn how to make your own lavender *extracted* oil, turn to page 190).

Taking the dried herb first: **sachets made of the dried herb are great to wrap sweaters and wool blankets in to keep away pesky moths**. I take a square piece of muslin, sew up the sides and stuff it full of dried lavender flowers, than sew it shut. (For additional "moth guard," I also place a few cedar blocks amongst the sweaters).

That same muslin sachet works in the bath as a scent-sational calmer-downer. Pour a hot bath and place the muslin sachet bag in the water, allowing it to steep like a giant tea. After the water is comfortable to the touch, soak for no longer than 30 minutes then go right to bed. This can do wonders for people who have **trouble sleeping due to nervous exhaustion or are unable to stop that endless "tape" in their head.** A lavender bath is also a fine idea for women who can't halt that **PMS** deal, too. The bath does wonders for **sunburn relief** (although, I'd certainly let the water cool considerably so you don't aggravate the burn!) And believe it or not, a lavender bath has been known to **stimulate the immune system.** Taking a lavender bath every other day has actually helped some people build up resistance to colds and infections while revving up their circulation. (Adding about eight drops of lavender essential oil really perks up this routine). Because of its natural antiseptic qualities, children in rural villages in France are regularly given lavender baths to keep them in good health. Those villagers may not be so far off the mark. Herbalists believe that lavender actually has the ability to **stimulate white blood cells which kill off the infection invaders**.

A strong infusion of dried lavender makes an excellent **douche for leucorrhea**. A potent brew would equal approximately one tablespoon of the dried herb steeped in one cup of very hot water. Allow to cool, making sure the mixture is covered completely when it is steeping.

Dried lavender sprays are a common sight when an interior decorator wants to inject a "country-fied" atmosphere. What they may not realize is that those dried flower arrangements hung around the house can act as a **bug repellent for flies and mosquitoes**.

While the dried herb is lovely, lavender pure essential oil is a much more portable way to enjoy this herb. Besides the fact that the oil is inexpensive, it is medicinally concentrated and can be used for lots of neat stuff. Replace the dried herbs in the muslin sachet with 10-15 drops of the lavender pure essential oil poured into the water *right before* you get in so the medicinal value within the herb doesn't evaporate with the scent. (By the way, lavender extracted oil also works well for this. In fact, you can substitute the extracted oil for the pure essential oil at any time).

Lavender essential oil is unique in the fact that it's one of the few distilled oils which can be safely poured onto the skin undiluted. Most essential oils are so strong that you risk burning or irritating the skin with a direct drop. However, don't let this "gentle-to-the-skin-fact" make you think that lavender oil isn't one tough trooper when it comes to fighting infection, pain or even rejuvenating dead skin. Consider this:

- Two or three drops of the pure essential oil on a nasty **oven burn** (applied *immediately*) will cut the pain, help prevent blistering, take out the heat within minutes and speed healing like nobody's business.
- One or two drops on a **minor cut or scrape** will kill harmful bacteria and speed healing.
- One or two drops on a **broken blister** will help the skin the heal faster. If the blister is on your hand, you can also use a lavender

oil and cold water soak for further relief. To do this, fill a bowl with two cups of cold tap water and add 10-20 drops of pure lavender essential oil. The essence will last for about 20 minutes before losing its medicinal strength.

- One drop on a **pimple** can start the healing process without the drying effects of medicated treatments.

- One or two drops on an **insect bite or bee/wasp sting** can reduce pain and swelling. (For a bee/wasp sting, you obviously have to take out the stinger first).

- One or two drops applied over a **tick** encourages the tick to back out of the skin, allowing you to pull it out faster. The strong antiseptic value of lavender pure essential oil also aids in disinfecting the area, just in case the tick is carrying any nasty infections.

- One drop on an on-coming **cold sore** can sometimes stop the full blown breakout. The pure essential oil often works better rather than the extracted oil.

- A whiff of the oil from the bottle, 3-5 drops placed on a cotton ball or one drop placed under the nose (not *in* it) can bring about calm in cases of **shock, hysteria, panic, dizziness and even bring back to life those who have fainted.** For this application, the pure essential oil is sometimes a better bet since it is more concentrated.

- Five to eight drops placed in a pot of hot water and inhaled deeply can **relieve coughs and stubborn chest congestion**.

- Several drops rubbed on the back of the neck and the base of the skull can gradually alleviate a **headache—especially those which start with a sharp pain at the base of the skull. Migraine** sufferers may also get relief if the lavender oil is used at the onset of the pain.

- Several drops rubbed into the nape of the neck can help reduce **throbbing hangover pain** provided you *also* lie down and rest.

- Two or three drops dropped onto the pillowcase can **promote a wonderful night's sleep** and has even been known to **prevent nightmares**.

- One drop in a baby's bath water helps to **soothe and stop an infant's crying**. It's important to *only put one drop of the lavender pure essential oil or lavender extracted oil in the water because more than that can irritate the infant's sensitive skin.*

- Two to three drops on a water-soaked washcloth and placed on the forehead can help to **reduce an adult's or child's fever and make it easier to get some rest**.
- Five to eight drops in a foot bath helps to **increase sluggish circulation in the feet and lower legs**.
- Four drops added to one tablespoon of sesame or safflower oil can be rubbed into **stretch marks** to smooth and even reduce them. That same combo can also be used as a gentle massage oil for **neuralgia or rheumatic pain**. Rub this blend on your tummy to **relieve period or PMS cramping**. Add two drops of chamomile essential oil (a bit more pricey) to the blend and you've got a natural lotion to **relieve pain from shingles**.
- The same massage oil is a marvelous calming rub to use on the **lower back for sciatic pain**.
- The massage oil can also be **rubbed into the chest when one is sick and can't get to sleep**.

The **mental/emotional response lavender tends to create is one of calmness, clarity and peace of mind**. Some aromatherapists say that diffusing lavender into a room **helps balance emotional instability, alleviate depression and counter feelings of suspicion**. However, they also warn that too much exposure to lavender can result in nausea. So, obviously, don't overdo a good thing or you could certainly defeat your purpose.

The only caution lavender carries is that in very high doses, it can be a uterine stimulant. For this reason, **pregnant women should be careful with both the dried herb and pure essential oil. Minimal exposure (i.e., one or two drops) is fine. However, if you are pregnant, do not douse yourself in the oil or drink more than one cup of the tea each day.**

Without a doubt, this herb—*especially* the oil—is a gentle giant in the plant kingdom. Maybe those ancient Romans weren't so crazy after all.

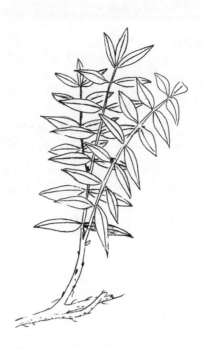

LICORICE—
A BEAUT OF A ROOT

Latin name: *Glycyrrhiza glabra*
Medicinal parts: the root
Forms: tea, dried root sticks

There is a time to live and a time to die.

And there's a time to cough.

It's usually when the first sign of cold weather creeps up faster than old underwear. Traditionally at the time of "The Cough" we are bombarded with commercials showing us what we can buy to "suppress that cough," "coat that cough," "kill that cough." Most over-the-counter preparations contain alcohol which can antagonize a cough and turn a person into two of the seven dwarfs: Sleepy and Dopey.

How grand it is to know that there is an herb which can ease a cough without putting you to sleep. In fact, this herb supports your system, giving you energy and stamina.

I'm talking about licorice root. I'm *not* talking about licorice candy. The candy contains sugar and that doesn't do the trick. Licorice root, though, has so much natural sweetness in it that it's roughly 50 times sweeter than sucrose. You can thank the multi-syllabic ingredient *glycyrrhizin* for that feat. Not only does that hard-to-pronounce word supply all the sweetness you'll ever need, it is also responsible for giving licorice root its **throat-coating, stomach-soothing, thirst-quenching, anti-inflammatory, anti-allergic, hormone-helping, adrenal gland boosting properties**. A big word with big results.

This root has history. The Egyptians buried sticks of licorice root deep in the tomb of King Tut, certain that it was a cure-all for what ails you. In the 5th century B.C., Hippocrates did his version of public relations for the root, telling how valuable it could be. The armies of Alexander the Great chewed on this gnarly root to keep up their strength and stamina while marching for long hours. In China, the dried root is still given to children to chew to help promote muscle growth.

Licorice root—taken in tea form—is an herb that truly deserves a place in today's history. Here are a few things it can do for you.

- *"The Cough"*—Licorice root tea sipped throughout the day can be a godsend for **itchy-scratchy coughs to the full-blown honking coughs**. Not only does the hot tea feel good going down, licorice's **anti-inflammatory ability** helps to reduce the irritation. In addition, licorice root tea will **break up congestion in the chest and loosen phlegm** which further relieves the cough. Don't be surprised if you start coughing up phlegm after several cups of licorice tea. That's the herb simply doing its job. But wait! There's more! Those sly lab scientists discovered a powerful *natural* antibiotic within the root called *triterpenoid glycyrrhetic acid* which kills existing and invading bacteria in the throat and throughout the body. Now, if this herb ain't a cough plant, I don't know what is! To enjoy the root tea, make a decoction by boiling one heaping teaspoon of the chopped dried root in 10 oz. of distilled water. You can drink up to four cups a day—sweetened with honey to coat the throat even more—to help suppress a cough and allow it to heal.

You can also make an old fashioned cough syrup out of the whole licorice root sticks or root sections. To make the syrup, follow the directions given on page 186.

- *"The Adrenal Glands"*—The glandular system needs to be kept clean and strong. The adrenal glands, especially, need support as well as a boost every five hours or so. The adrenals, which lie directly on the top of the kidneys, can become swollen and tender when trying to process too many toxins. Licorice tea can help bring the adrenals back to life, producing more adrenalin and, thus, energy. Hypoglycemics can really benefit from the herb because of its high sweetness content which translates into a dose of blood sugar. Some signs that your adrenals may be overtaxed include bouts of low energy (especially around 3:00 in the afternoon when many folks crave a "pick-me-up" sweet treat or cup of coffee), oversleeping but not feeling rested, dark circles and/or bags under the eyes, the inability to fight off allergies, hormone deficiency, skin disorders, arthritic conditions and a general feeling of being run down. It is always best to check with a doctor or herbal practitioner if you feel your condition is chronic.

- *"Asthma relief"*—While licorice is certainly no magic remedy for serious asthma sufferers, it does have the ability to reduce the congestion that can often times bring on an attack. Boil three licorice roots—whole or grated—in one pint of distilled water for twenty minutes. Strain and sip throughout the day. Those with asthma should also avoid mucus-forming foods such as red meat, eggs, bread and dairy products.

- *"Hay fever & Allergies"*—Licorice root tea helps to build up the body's resistance to allergens. Once again, diet is extremely important. Synthetic sugar and dairy products clog the system which depletes the body's ability to fight off the incoming allergic poisons. Replacing sugar with fresh fruits and vegetables as well as incorporating more vitamin C, calcium and magnesium into your system can aid in building up resistance to allergies. The licorice root tea can then work more effectively in combating the evil intruders. For allergies, it's best to take only one cup per day for a six day period, cease taking the tea for one week and then resume for six days.

- *"Arthritis-soothing"*—I feel like a broken record but once again, DIET must be considered. Those nasty sugars and milk products should be avoided. The **anti-inflammatory properties** of licorice root result from its ability to stimulate two steroids: cortisone and aldosterone. When activated, these steroids act as soothing cushions for the inflamed joints. Two to three cups per day are sufficient. Take for three days on and three days off, see how you feel and then resume.

- *"Ulcers"*—A cup or two of licorice root tea each day for up to five days has shown remarkable results in soothing peptic ulcers and stomach irritations. It appears to spread a protective gel over the stomach wall which absorbs acid and creates a more pH-balanced environment. In addition, licorice calms the stomach and intestines, helping to reduce spasms in the large intestine. Chinese scientists have even gone so far as to say that licorice actually "cures" peptic ulcers if the tea is taken at the beginning of an attack. If you wait until the ulcer becomes too inflamed, say the Chinese, the herb doesn't work as effectively.

- *"Hormone-helping"*—Licorice is a natural source of the female hormone estrogen which makes it a fabulous support tea for **post hysterectomy care**. It's also helpful for the female body during menopause. **However, women who suffer from PMS should not use licorice during that time since the herb can cause water retention**.

- *"Public Speaker Tea"*—If you are someone who spends a great deal of the day talking, sipping a cup or two of licorice tea throughout the day can help coat and soothe your throat and buffer it against that **"scratchy-catch-in-the-throat"** feeling. If you can't make the tea, you can chew on a stick of licorice root, pulverizing the meaty center between your teeth and swallowing the liquid. Others might think you're chewing on a tree branch, but you'll know better.

- *"Staying Alert"*—I've used licorice root tea so many times when I needed to stay alert during a long day. Because licorice root supports the adrenal system, sipping on a thermos of licorice root tea throughout the day is a great way to maintain energy without that "caffeine buzz."

There are several cautions with licorice. **If you suffer from high blood pressure, *do not* use licorice root tea**. The increased production of aldosterone in the body can raise blood pressure. **You should also avoid the herb if you suffer from rapid heart beats. If you are taking digoxin-based drugs, avoid the herb. *Do not* take licorice tea for any longer than three weeks at a time since it can sap potassium from the body**. I usually drink the tea for 10 days then take two weeks off and see how I feel. **Licorice tea has a tendency over time to cause weight gain—mostly due to** water retention. If you are on a weight-loss program, I'd stay away from the tea except on a limited basis. **If, on the other hand, you are trying to gain weight, and you don't fall into any of the no-no categories mentioned above, give it a try.** Finally, **if you suffer from edema, stay away from licorice tea since its water-retention capabilities will only make the problem worse. Pregnant women can drink licorice tea *in small amounts* after the first trimester as long as they are not experiencing edema. However, since edema is often common during the last trimester of pregnancy, it is best to refrain from the root at that time.**

When used correctly and carefully, this beaut of a root can do more than you ever imagined.

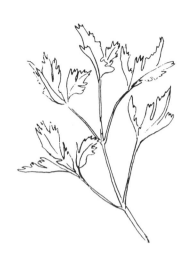

PARSLEY—THE GARNISH WITH GUSTO

Latin name: Petroselinum sativum
Medicinal parts: plant, seeds
Forms: tea, pure essential oil

I'm guilty of it and so are you. You see the parsley on the plate—that colorful splash of green—and spin it around the dish. You don't eat it—heavens no—it's decoration. Like streamers. They add a decorative spark to a party but you don't eat them. No, leave that parsley right there. It's just for color.

Wrong!

If people knew how great parsley really is, they'd fall down on their knees in thanks. This weedy piece of "decoration" is **one of** *the* **best vitamin-filled-mineral-rich-iron-laden tonic herbs available**. The best part is you don't have to search high and low for it—the darn stuff is everywhere! And thank goodness for that because there are case studies where parsley has literally saved someone's life.

It's strange that an herb with such life-giving abilities would be known in legend as more of a "death" herb. It was planted on Greek graves and, thanks to Greek mythology, was considered to be bad luck for a soldier if he saw it before going into battle. In other words, it's the last thing the battle cook would serve to add color to the plate. Actually, parsley could have been what those soldiers needed before fighting the enemy. It is *loaded* with vitamins A, C, E, K, B$_2$, B$_3$ and folic acid. There are *30,000 I.U.* of vitamin A in each ounce! And there's three times more vitamin C than in a glass of citrus juice. Looking for iron? Parsley has more iron in its little spindle than *any other* green leafy vegetable.

Parsley is great for many ailments. However, it gets the awards for its **diuretic capabilities**.

As a diuretic, parsley is at the top of its herbal class. It is this ability which has saved lives—especially in cases where urine was backing up and poisoning the kidneys and liver. Parsley does not allow salt to be re-absorbed into body tissues and literally forces debris out of the kidneys, liver and bladder. With parsley tea it's important to remember that—unlike most other herbs—**one must drink a lot of the green stuff to start the flushing action**. This in itself might be a task since the taste of parsley tea—especially fresh parsley tea—has a very "green bouquet" to it. It's not bad tasting, it's just kind of grassy. Instead of the usual one teaspoon to 8 oz. of water routine, combine one heaping tablespoon of the root or leaves or one handful of the fresh plant to a pint of boiling water. Cover and steep for 20 minutes, strain and then drink the pint in large gulps.

Parsley tea can work especially well **when urination is painful or sparse due to an enlarged prostate**. Of course, don't fool around with an enlarged prostate. Go to the doctor, get an opinion and find out what else can be done to help the condition—either with herbs or medically. Parsley tea, in this case, is simply a temporary way to alleviate urinary discomfort.

Chronic and acute bladder infections have also been helped—sometimes within two days—by massive cups of parsley tea. Often times, though, where infection is present, it is best to combine parsley with other herbs that are infection-fighters (such as echinacea or garlic). Adding equal parts of the herbs buchu, juniper berries and uva ursi can also work to cleanse the urinary tract and kill infection.

The second biggie for parsley is **bringing on a menstrual period**. Mind you, it may take three to four hot cups of parsley tea to produce this phenomena. As well as stimulating the uterine muscles, several hot cups of parsley tea also give a woman a healthy dose of vitamins and minerals. For this reason, a hot cup of parsley tea can also do wonders for quelling **menstrual cramps or cramping due to an upset or nervous stomach**.

Which brings me to **digestion**. ("Ah," you're saying, "that's why they stuck it on the plate"). Yes, that gentle sprig of parsley eaten raw or made into a tea can do wonders for your digestive juices. Not only does it quell **indigestion,** it actually **helps your body assimilate food and minerals**. And it **sweetens the breath**! "Nature's chlorophyll" **dowses the pungent odors of garlic and onion**. And gas! Did I mention gas? If that meal has you **belching**, simply chew on that sprig until the juice just oozes out and then swallow. You can also make a cup of parsley tea to help dissipate **gas pains**. Use the basic formula of one teaspoon of the dried herb or two teaspoons of the fresh herb to 8 oz. of hot distilled water.

Since parsley gives your bladder a jump start and your kidneys a thorough wash, it makes sense that it can also **clear the liver of toxins**. The same copious amounts of tea that are used as a diuretic should be used for the liver. However, if you have any chronic liver condition, for heaven's sake seek professional help before self-medicating. Too much dumping of toxic garbage could set your progress back instead of helping you to move forward.

This all-around tonic has also shown promise when it comes to helping folks suffering from **arthritis and rheumatism**. Because it encourages a breakdown of toxins and acids that meet and greet each other in the joints, a strong cup of parsley root tea, taken once or twice a day, may bring relief.

The tea also **soothes bronchial passages** and can be your friend if you suffer from **asthma**. While we're on the breathing front, **chronic sinus congestion** has been helped a great deal by taking 3-4 cups of parsley tea each day or two tablets of garlic and parsley every four hours for six days straight. If, after six days, you still don't have relief, see your doctor or holistic practitioner.

As a **blood-building tea** for those folks who are **recuperating from an illness**, parsley can't be beat. The best way to expel the iron-rich nutrients is by drinking parsley juice. To really perk up the drink, add two parts fresh spinach to one part parsley. I'll admit, it's a drink that has to grow on you and might be unpleasant for some people. If that's the case and you still want to benefit from parsley's vitalizing properties, drop a few slices of the parsley root into plain vegetable or meat broth and enjoy.

Got an **allergy**? Parsley tea might be your ticket to sneeze-free living. A study showed that parsley inhibits the secretion of histamine, which is a chemical your body produces that triggers the allergy attack. Look on parsley as a natural antihistamine without the groggy side-effects.

Researchers are also looking into the possible benefits of parsley as a **diabetes** aid. I know someone with diabetes who drinks parsley tea regularly (along with other herbs his holistic doctor prescribed). He feels that the parsley has given him more energy and renewed strength. Once again, check with your doctor or an holistic practitioner.

Externally, parsley is equally as impressive. Make a poultice out of the fresh or dried herb and apply it to an **insect bite or sting** for pain relief and reduced swelling. The fresh juice rubbed on the skin gives you a safe, non-toxic **insect repellent. Swollen glands**? Dip a cloth in the hot tea and lay it against the area, taking care to keep the cloth warm. And the bruised leaves steeped in cider vinegar and **applied to swollen breasts will help reduce the swelling as well as dry up mother's milk**. You can also use parsley essential oil in a massage oil for this task. Combine no more than five drops of the pure essential parsley oil to one ounce of almond oil or apricot kernel oil and massage the breast gently. However, be aware that while the swelling is reduced, the breast milk may begin to dry up. If you still want to use this parsley massage oil to reduce breast swelling but don't want to dry up the milk, simply massage the breast with the oil and pay close attention to any signs of milk depletion. If you notice any loss, stop using the massage oil.

Yes, there are cautions and they are all biggies. Even though parsley has shown itself to help pull people through severe kidney disease, **it's not recommended if there is a serious infection. Because the tea is used to induce menstruation, pregnant women should NEVER drink the tea. Chewing on that one decorative sprig, however, is fine. Don't go out picking parsley in the wild because it** looks just like hemlock—you know, the stuff that promotes the "Big Sleep." Cultivate it in your garden or window box to play it safe.

I just know that the next time you come face to face with that winsome splash of green on your dinner plate, you'll think twice before scooting it across your dish.

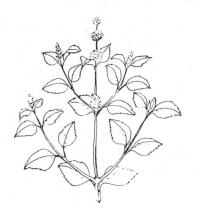

THE POWER'S IN THE PEPPERMINT

Latin name: Mentha piperita
Medicinal parts: leaves
Forms: tea, pure essential oil, extracted oil

You've seen the commercial. The woman is standing in her kitchen after coming home from work. She's surrounded by a flock of screaming kids. Her husband opens the door and asks "What's for dinner, honey?" The walls start to cave in. Her face warps as though she's looking into a fun house mirror. Then you hear a deep-voice say: "Molly McDonald—Tension headache #153. When the head starts to pound, you need powerful, *fast* relief. Reach for *Peppermint???*"

Don't I *wish* they'd say that! Instead they hawk another brand of pain relief that will knock you into a dull stupor and often add more problems such as stomach upset, nausea or dizziness. No thanks.

Whenever I get **headaches**—whether it's from eyestrain or good ol' stress—I do three things. First, and most importantly, I stop doing whatever is causing the headache. Secondly, I bring out my little bottle of peppermint essential oil and dab a drop on each temple as well as a drop or two on the nape of my neck. And thirdly, if I can, I lie down for 10-15 minutes, close my eyes and relax.

Hey, when your head starts to pound, your body is trying to tell you something. "I'm on overload!" it's screaming and it creates a headache to get the message to your brain that your body is out of balance. In my opinion, covering up the headache with pain killing capsules are a last resort. Next time you feel the pressure and the pound of a headache, just for kicks, try a more natural approach with peppermint. You can use the herb in a multitude of ways including the traditional tea, the pure essential oil, baths and cooling and calming compresses (fomentations).

Two to three drops of peppermint pure essential oil, when applied to the temples and nape of neck, provide almost instant cooling relief from headaches. For a real "cooling sensation," dot a moistened washcloth with no more than three drops of peppermint pure essential oil. Place the washcloth across your forehead and lie down for 15-20 minutes. Be careful to not get the washcloth near your eyes or they will start to sting and water something fierce. If this happens, simply wash your eyes with cool water and dip the washcloth in cold water to rinse out the oil. Replace the washcloth across your forehead and continue to relax.

You can achieve the same, yet milder effect, using a tea fomentation—i.e., dipping a washcloth in a strong cool peppermint tea blend and laying it across your forehead. To generate a double dose of headache relief, couple the washcloth bit with a hot cup of peppermint tea. Make an infusion by combining 1 teaspoon of the dried herb or two teaspoons of the fresh leaves to an 8 oz. of boiling water, cover and steep for 10-15 minutes, strain and enjoy.

One consideration here: if you're buying peppermint tea in the convenient bag form, read the label and make sure that *only* peppermint leaves are in the mixture. Sometimes herbal tea manufacturers add other herbs such as orange blossom and lemon peel. While these are certainly fine herbs, it's better to drink 100% peppermint tea in order to get the full effect. As with all infusions, NEVER boil the leaves. Boiling the leaves drains out most of the volatile oils and herbal agents that are contained within the plant.

Peppermint tea has had quite the reputation through the herbal ages. Some old European herbal books even touted it as the tea to drink "when you wanteth to conceive a male child." I don't think I'd put that kind of pressure on the mint. But, believe me, this herb has plenty of *proven* power to back it up. For example, research has found that peppermint tea **can inhibit and kill over 30 micro-organisms**. These micro-organisms (or "bugs" to the novice) are known to cause everything from the **Asian flu virus** and **mumps** to **herpes simplex** and **candida** (**which can bring on yeast infections**).

Regarding **herpes simplex**, two cups of warm peppermint tea taken daily during a flare-up, have really helped to halt the cold sore's growth. One or two drops of the essential oil on a cotton ball and applied directly to the **cold sore** for two to three minutes have also proven to be a winner in speeding the healing. The trick is to get the peppermint tea into your body as soon as you notice the first sign of herpes and dot that essential oil on the sore before it gets out of hand. This treatment may not work for everyone—especially if your body is loaded down with toxins. But, hey, it's worth a try.

Probably one of peppermint tea's most popular uses is as a **digestive aid**. No wonder that many restaurants offer you a peppermint candy after your meal. Of course, while candy is dandy, the tea is a better bet, especially when one cup is taken an hour after a meal. The herb will help stimulate your liver and keep your digestive juices flowing. If the tea is also drunk *before* heavy meals, you might be able to avoid **gas pains**.

Peppermint tea tends to be the "stopping tea" in that it can **stop or reduce heavy menstrual flow** as well as **reduce or stop the flow of mother's milk**. Obviously, if these two tricks aren't something you want your body to experience, you may want to take it easy on your peppermint tea consumption.

A cup of peppermint tea in the evening can sometimes be the ticket for people who deal with **daily stress and have trouble winding down**. However, often this herb reacts just the opposite and can jump start your body. It also has a tendency to jump-start your mind and helps to get those mental juices flowing. For this reason, it's a great tea for **weary business travelers** to try when they've been traveling all day and need to shine for that late-night dinner or meeting. A cup or two before the engagement can give you a nicer wake up call than caffeine or chocolate.

Peppermint tea perks up those folks who **faint** or experience **dizzy spells**. In this case, you can use a stronger brew—up to a tablespoon of the leaves to 8 oz. of hot distilled water—to get the body back on track. (I've also found that when you soak a cotton ball with 3-5 drops of peppermint pure essential oil and breathe in the aroma, it helps to relieve the symptoms even more).

Because peppermint tastes good, kids tend to be more willing to try it. Sometimes a cup of hot peppermint tea—sipped not gulped—is all it takes to **soothe a child when they've had a minor physical or emotional upset**. However, **peppermint tea and essential oil should *not* be used for children under the age of two**.

Peppermint tea is fantastic but I've got to tell you, the pure essential oil is even better. I like it so much I carry a 1/2 oz. bottle in my purse all the time. It only takes a drop or two of the pure essential oil to fully appreciate the power of the herb. Sometimes, the aroma is so strong it can make your eyes tear. If this becomes a problem, you can always make an extracted oil from the fresh or dried plant. (Turn to page 190 to learn how to make extracted oil).

Peppermint oil really stirs up the senses as well as the circulation. Because of this, the essential oil works well for anyone who needs to **concentrate and stay alert**. It works great for students who need that extra aromatic boost to keep them **focused and awake**. Independent studies have shown that when students either sniffed the pure essential oil of peppermint or diffused the oil into the room, they retained 25-30% more of the information. The best way to take in peppermint's perky scent is to put one or two drops of the pure essential oil onto your palm, then quickly rub your palms together. Cup your hands and bring them up to your nose, taking in a deep breath. Alternate breaths through your nose and mouth no more than three times. *You do not want to overdo this little exercise since it has been known to jump start the circulation and heart rather quickly. It can also cause lightheadedness and burning in the eyes.* So, please, don't abuse the essential oil's power.

There's a whole lot o' menthol in the mint and it's jam packed in the concentrated essential oil. Some peppermint researchers found that the menthol content makes the oil **extremely antiseptic**. That means that when you get a **minor kitchen burn** or a **superficial scrape**, a couple drops of the essential oil can help sterilize the skin as well as cool the pain on contact.

Sinus congestion can also be relieved by either trying a steam inhalation with the oil (see page 192 for details), rubbing the oil between your palms as mentioned above, or rubbing a drop of peppermint oil under each nostril (not *in* the nose, *under* the nose!) However, only depend upon peppermint for several days since, because of the high menthol content, prolonged use can eventually dry up the sensitive skin in and around the nose.

This portable peppermint oil is great to take on camp outs or picnics where there are sure to be **mosquitoes** sharing the air space. Yeah, it's that menthol again that repels those flying critters.

A massage oil (made by combining 15-20 drops of the essential oil or extracted oil with one ounce of sweet almond or sunflower oil) is a wonderful rub for nursing mothers who need relief from **milk congestion in the breast. However, since the tea has been known to reduce or even stop the flow of mother's milk, take care that you don't over-stimulate the breast with this massage oil. The oil will penetrate into the tissues and help alleviate congestion. Once the congestion is taken care of, stop using the massage oil. If you notice any sudden reduction or stoppage in breast milk, cease using the massage oil.**

A few drops of the essential oil in a gallon of tap water makes a **stimulating hair rinse**. A peppermint bath is a wonderful way to cool off on a hot summer day. It's also a good bath when you have a nasty **poison ivy/oak rash**. Check out page 151 to find out all about the peppermint bath.

On the emotional/mental front, peppermint pure essential oil is **very uplifting** and tends to **spark enthusiasm** when people are around the aroma. Some aromatherapists claim that peppermint essential oil may even help you gain better **discernment** and be more **decisive.**

There are cautions to peppermint—both in the tea and oil form. **Don't overdose on peppermint in any form**. The tea can be very stimulating to the body—especially if you use the fresh leaves. Some herbalists suggest taking the herbal tea medicinally for only four days (at two cups maximum each day) waiting seven days and then repeating only if you feel you need it. **Pregnant women need to be cautious about the tea and essential oil since large doses can stimulate the uterine muscles. Do not use the essential oil during the first trimester. After that, only use it sparingly and only if you feel you need it. If** you are pregnant and want to drink peppermint tea, cut the normal recipe in half (i.e., one half teaspoon to 8 oz. of hot distilled water) and only steep the tea for 2-3 minutes. In addition, if you are pregnant, do not drink more than one cup of peppermint tea each day and for no longer than two days in a row with seven days off in between.

As for the pure essential oil, remember not to overdo it when inhaling the aromatic vapors. The oil is extremely concentrated. Not only can prolonged use affect the sensitive mucous membranes but your nervous system can be thrown into a tailspin.

Also, there is a big difference between American-processed essential oils and European-processed essential oils. The European distilled oils have a different filtering system which makes many of them pure enough to be taken by drop *internally*. In fact, many essential oils distilled in Germany are expressly made as an internal medicinal essential oil. However, American-processed essential oils are *not* made to be taken internally as the labels should note. Because many essential oils are costly to distill, some American manufacturers use petroleum-based solvents to extract the oil. Others steam distill, but cut the oil with mineral oil to make the product more affordable. For this reason, do not take any American-processed pure essential oils internally in *any* form—that means not diluted in water, not on a sugar cube—just not on anything. If you have European-processed pure essential oils, only take those internally with a doctor's permission *and only* if the bottle says explicitly that the oil can be used internally.

Yeah, peppermint is known worldwide as one powerhouse herb. Now if we could just get that poor woman with the screaming kids, the demanding husband and the warped face to brew up a cup of peppermint tea.

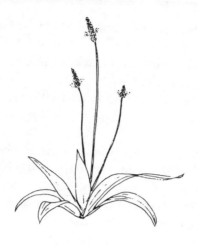

PLANTAIN & SIMPLE

Latin name: *Plantago lanceolata and*
            Plantago major
Medicinal parts: the plant
Forms: fresh plant, tea, ointment

Walking down a friend's driveway, I spotted a lively stalk of plantain poking its head between the cracks. "Ah," I said in herbal awe, "you started a little herb garden." My friend peered down at the crack, curled her lip and said, "That's not an herb! That's plantain! I hate the stuff! You can't get rid of it!" I was going to tell her how lucky she was to have such a great little herb peeking through the driveway, but I don't think she would have believed me.

The one thing she was right about is that plantain is a mighty strong little weed. Call it "The Hearty Herb," call it "The Stubborn Herb," whatever you choose, it's a tough puppy. Those wagon-rollin' pioneers might have called it "The Well-Trampled Herb" because plantain grew freely from the wagon ruts they carved into the earth. And no matter how many wheels crushed it or button top boots kicked it, the stuff never died. In fact, plantain is so resilient, it'll grow where nothing else will. What a trooper.

Thanks to those happy homesteaders, plantain covers most of this country. It seems that the seeds become quite sticky when wet and attach themselves to everything from shoes to wagon wheels to hooves. So the frontier folk might have picked up a plantain seed in

Kansas on the heel of their shoe and "planted" it in Colorado one month later.

Hearty, yes, and very helpful too. In fact, plantain is one herb I would put at the top of my list.

There are two different species: narrowleaf plantain and what they call broadleaf plantain. However, they each have the same medicinal value. This is an herb which truly *works better when used fresh out of the ground especially when it comes to wounds, rashes and insect bites.* If you are planning on collecting plantain fresh from the ground, consider two things:

1. Make sure you collect it when the plant is in bloom and,

2. Make sure you're picking plantain!

Many people have gotten plantain mixed up with various lilies and even the dangerous green hellebore (yikes!) so know exactly what you're plantain pickin'!

Plantain has a reputation for being one of the best remedies for **coughs, lung congestion, hoarseness and anything where excessive mucus is a problem**. Many families depend upon plantain tea or homemade syrup to get them through the night when coughing fits get out of hand. To make the tea, make an infusion, adding one heaping teaspoon of the dried herb to 8 oz. of hot distilled water. Feel free to drink up to three cups of plantain tea a day when those really stubborn, mucus-laden coughs get the better of you.

To make the syrup, the *fresh leaves* work best. However, if you only have dried leaves, that'll work. Chop up four heaping handfuls of freshly washed leaves or two handfuls of dried leaves and put them in a pot. Add 4-6 cups of distilled water. Heat the mixture very gently, stirring continually. Keep stirring until the liquid is half its original volume. This can take anywhere from 30 minutes to an hour depending upon the heat source you are using. Once the volume is reduced, take the pot off the stove, strain the liquid and then measure it. Now, double that number. That is the amount of honey you need to add to the mixture. (In other words, if you end up with two cups of plantain tea, add four cups of honey). Gradually stir in the honey and then bring the mixture just to a boil. Turn off the heat and add a one-inch square piece of fresh ginger root. The ginger root helps to strengthen the effectiveness of the syrup as well as give it a longer storage life. Pour the syrup into a bottle with a cork stopper and shake the bottle each time you use it. Take up to four tablespoons of the syrup each hour whenever a hacking cough starts to hammer on you. If it is kept refrigerated, the syrup can last up to one month.

Since plantain is such a lung-related herb, it works well for those people (especially kids) who have **chronic lung congestion**. For this ailment, the dosage is one cup of plantain tea each morning using a scant teaspoon of the dried leaves to 8 oz. of distilled water. Continue with the tea for three weeks, then take 10 days off to give your body a rest.

The other big time use for plantain is as a **wound-cut-sting-insect bite remedy**. They have actually done scientific experiments where fresh, mashed plantain leaves (either the broadleaf or narrowleaf will do) were immediately applied to wounds, cuts and insect bites and within 30 minutes, the pain and inflammation were greatly reduced. And since plantain is also a fabulous **coagulator of blood**, if there was any bleeding related to the above, the herb helped slow the flow.

With stings and insect bites, plantain has been shown to draw out the insect's poison before it can cause major discomfort. The same has been shown with **dog bites (even rabid dog bites)** where fresh crushed and moistened plantain leaves were *immediately* applied to the dog bite as the patient was being taken to the emergency room. The poultice not only prevented any further poisoning, it also worked to pull out much of the infection.

I've seen this incredible poultice work its wonder within minutes. One summer, I visited a friend on her farm. The house sat in a field of green grass, rich with herbal weeds—including plantain.

One day, my friend was reaching into her purse when she let out a loud scream. It seems a wasp was hiding inside one of the pockets and took the opportunity to sting her index finger. Within seconds, her finger started to turn red and swell. I immediately ran outside to where the plantain was growing. I snapped off three leaves, layered them on top of one another and gently bit into them to bring out the juices. I then wrapped the three moistened leaves around my friend's finger and told her to hold it in place for 15 minutes. She looked at me as though I was one card short of a full deck, but agreed to do as I said. Within 10 minutes, she suddenly realized her finger wasn't on fire anymore. Five minutes later, she unwrapped the plantain and saw that the redness was completely gone. The only sign of the sting was a pinpoint sized red dot. A couple more fresh, moistened plantain leaves took care of that complaint within 30 minutes. To say plantain is an amazing herb is putting it mildly in my book.

If you find yourself in a similar situation (i.e., a wasp or bee sting), and can identify the plantain plant, remember that the *fresh,* lightly chewed up leaves work the best. Chewing the leaves is essential since the juice within the leaves holds the healing punch. And don't just pat the sting or bite with the wet leaves, firmly press the plantain poultice against the inflamed area and hold it there for 10-15 minutes.

Mother Nature has plopped plantain in the most convenient spots. Believe it or not, if you're out in the woods and you brush up against the **poison oak/ivy** or feel the bite of **stinging nettle**, stop dead in your tracks and look around the area carefully. Within eyesight, you will notice that plantain, yellow dock, mullein and/or hounds tongue is growing nearby. All of these plants—but most specifically plantain—can be moistened with saliva or water, crushed and applied to the affected area for quick relief. The sooner you apply the plantain the better when it comes to poison ivy/oak and nettle. When used immediately, I have found that the rash/burn dissipates within 15 minutes of applying the freshly moistened plantain leaves.

Since fresh plantain is the most effective form of the plant, I make a 2 oz. jar of the ointment out of the *fresh plant* to keep around the house during the months when plantain is not available. I have found the ointment is the second best choice to using the fresh plant. Unfortunately, the dried leaves made into a wet poultice don't cut it in this category. To learn how to make this very easy and important first-aid ointment, turn to page 188 and look under the "Ointment/Salve" section.

As a **wound healer**, plantain is considered superior. In addition to coagulating blood, plantain tea and ointment have been known to close up even the most **stubborn sores that refuse to mend**. For "old wounds" such as **foot or leg ulcers,** herbalists suggest taking the tea internally and using *fresh leaf* poultices externally on a daily basis. One could even wash the wound in a plantain bath using a cup of fresh leaves to a bucket of hot water. Let the mixture *cool* and soak the area you want to treat in the tea for up to 30 minutes. The cooling sensation of plantain is actually quite calming. After patting the wound dry, apply a mashed and slightly moistened poultice of fresh leaves to the wound and loosely bandage with breathable gauze. Leave on until the poultice is almost dry and then follow up with another wet poultice or the plantain ointment. Chronic wounds that did not respond to any kind of treatment have been known to perk up and mend with this natural aid. This same procedure also works for **skin eruptions and rashes** that won't go away.

When combining the external poultice with the internal intake of tea, you get a double whammy effect, *especially* when **blood poisoning** is involved. A freshly-mashed plantain poultice pressed into the area that is showing signs of blood poisoning can help to pull out the pain and, sometimes, the poison. Those tell-tale red streaks are *nothing* to fool around with, mind you, but plantain can be a wonderful stop-gap, natural first aid when you are out in the boonies and far from medical assistance.

There's even a rumor that placing fresh plantain leaves in the bottom of your shoes will **prevent blisters during long walks**. And if you already have blisters on your feet? Well, some herbalists swear that plantain leaves pressed firmly against the sole of the foot will **draw out the blister** and help it to heal quickly. Sounds strange? Maybe. But if it works, who has the last laugh?

I think it's pretty amazing how this "bothersome weed" can be plucked from the ground and put into action at a moment's notice. It may be considered "just a nasty weed" to some. But to others who have seen what it can do, it's the wisest weed on the block.

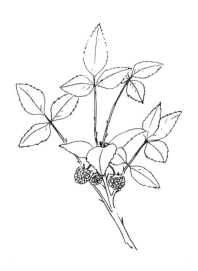

RALLY 'ROUND RED RASPBERRY LEAF

Latin name: *Rubus strigosus & Rubus idaeus*
Medicinal parts: leaves
Forms: tea

I remember picking red raspberries in the summertime when I was a kid. I always thought you had to go through a lot of trouble just to get a piece of fruit that was smaller than a quarter. I also didn't care for the prickly stems that held the berries prisoner until someone like myself risked a lifetime of scars just to disengage a piece of teeny fruit. Little did I know back then that the raspberry's deep green leaves held the secret that folk doctors and midwives had already discovered hundreds of years ago.

Which is: red raspberry leaves are **the best all-around tonic for pregnant women**. There are other herbs that help during pregnancy, but red raspberry leaf is sort of the king of the jungle, the foremost foliage, the premiere plant, you get the point.

Before I proceed, it's important to know that many herbs are considered forbidden during pregnancy. **While red raspberry is indicated for pregnant women, I must advise that if you're pregnant—or even planning to conceive—you** need to check with a holistic practitioner to make sure your individual body chemistry can tolerate this herb.

That said, red raspberry contains vitamins A, B, C, G and E as well as healthy doses of calcium, phosphorus and iron. All these nutrients play a major role in helping to not only **prevent miscarriages but ease the eventual delivery**.

Red raspberry is an astringent which means it has the ability to draw together tissue, muscles, skin, etc. During pregnancy, the tea gently tones the uterine and pelvic muscles which help to prepare the body to give birth. Because of the massive hormonal changes going on during pregnancy, it's easy for many women to lose a lot of necessary minerals and vitamins that feed both fetus and mother. Taking red raspberry tea helps to flood the system with healing and soothing nourishment.

There are a lot of opinions in the herb world as to when a pregnant woman should start drinking red raspberry tea. Some herbalists say one cup of the tea should be drunk each day before conception and continued daily until four weeks after giving birth. Others in the herb field say that high doses of the tea should absolutely be avoided during the first trimester; however, one cup of the tea should be drunk each day during the last two to three months of pregnancy, continuing until a couple weeks after giving birth to help the uterus return to normal. Obviously, there are clashes of opinion. For this reason, I strongly suggest consulting with an herbalist or holistic doctor who knows your medical history. If it checks out for you, the suggested way to drink red raspberry tea during pregnancy is to take one cup one half hour before either lunch or dinner.

If red raspberry does work out for you, you may discover some other interesting things the tea can do for you after giving birth. For example, when the tea is drunk daily from right after labor and for three days afterward, the astringent effect helps **after-pains, minimizes uterine swelling and cuts down on postpartum bleeding**. Another nifty effect you may encounter if you drink the tea right *before* labor and for several days thereafter is that **breast milk flow increases as well as becomes more enriched**.

Those little berries also can do a bang-up job against fighting **anemia**—a problem both pregnant and "non-pregnant" people combat. Once again, that powerful chorus of vitamins and minerals are part of the "magic." However, don't overdo on the fruit since they can cause one to become a little on the acidic side of happy.

Speaking of having babies, once that bundle of joy pops out, he or she might experience **diarrhea**. Red raspberry leaf tea can come to the rescue again as a wonderful, sweet-tasting alternative to those nasty, over-the-counter formulas. The secret is to *serve the tea cold* after simmering 1/2 oz. of the dried leaves in 1/2 pint of water for 20 minutes. Strain the leaves and let the tea sit until cool. Give it to the baby in small measured spoonfuls (i.e., no more than one teaspoon at a time every 10 minutes) rather than sticking it in a bottle and letting them gulp it down. Give no more than 1/2 oz. of the cold tea to a baby during an eight hour period.

This raspberry "run-remedy" also can work for adults, except use 1 oz. of the herb to 1/2 pint of water. Adults, too, need to slowly sip the cold tea which can be drunk up to three times a day (i.e., three 8 oz. cups three times a day). The only consideration here is that you must make sure that the diarrhea is not caused by something more serious—such as food poisoning, infection or parasites. If any of these conditions are the root of the problem, you need to address them specifically with herbs that help kill infection. (Herbs that fall into this category would be echinacea and garlic). If you just treat the diarrhea and don't get to the root of the problem (the infection), you won't stop the source of the intestinal disorder. It's like trying to clear a clogged drain by pulling out debris from the opening of the pipe and not reaming all the way to the source of the block. Visual, yes, but you get the drift now, don't you?

Still on the female front, red raspberry tea has been used for eons by women who wish to **decrease a heavy menstrual flow**. The herb's astringent action acts like a big sponge as it gently contracts the tissues and halts menstrual flooding. However, while red raspberry can slam the flood gates, it will not stop a period which makes it a kind and gentle herb. It is important to mention that if you experience continuous flooding during your period which lasts longer than five days, see your doctor immediately.

Red raspberry is not just the "pregnant" or "female" herb. Men (and anyone not pregnant) can take it. In fact, it's another one of those herbs that should be kept on the shelf all the time. Why? Because it is also considered a fabulous tea for the **cold and flu** season.

Good ol' Dr. John R. Christopher—considered by many to have been the main man when it came to herbs and their many uses—touted red raspberry leaf tea as the only thing standing between you and getting well. The blood making and nutrient qualities of red raspberry make it a one-stop-shop-herb for feeding and rejuvenating a sick body.

It works like this. Upon feeling the cold or flu coming on, immediately stop eating all solid foods and beverages. Prepare several quarts of red raspberry tea and drink only that for the first 24 hours. Figure mixing one ounce of the herb to every pint of distilled water. Of course, wash down the tea with additional supplements such as vitamin B, C, A and E to completely overload your body with flu-fighting allies. By the next day, you should see a vast improvement in how you feel and can introduce chicken broth or a baked potato into your diet (no butter, of course, on the potato).

Continue with several quarts of red raspberry leaf tea for up to three days—even if you're back to feeling in tip-top shape. The tea will do an **A-1 cleansing job on your liver and act as a tonic for the whole system**. I know this might sound like a harsh way to combat a cold, but if you're serious about getting well and not having to deal with the lingering effects of the flu, it's worth missing a few filling meals. And if you also happen to have a pesky problem with **high blood pressure**, you should see that drop like an iron ball after three days of drinking red raspberry tea.

There is also a great red raspberry formula I use as both a rejuvenating tonic after an illness and a "Spring Tonic" to recharge my body after winter. The herbs are as follows:

Red Raspberry	1 teaspoon
Red Clover	1 teaspoon
Nettle	1 teaspoon
Alfalfa	1/2 teaspoon
Horsetail	1/2 teaspoon
Cleavers	1/2 teaspoon
Parsley	1/2 teaspoon

Combine the herbs into a quart jar. Fill the jar with very hot water and put the lid on tightly. Shake the jar vigorously every few minutes. After 15 minutes, strain 8 oz. of the tea into a cup, replacing the soggy herbs back into the quart jar. I drink this tea mixture a cup at a time throughout the day. By the fourth cup, it's going to be strong since the herbs will have been steeping longer. You can drink the tea cold, however, if you want to re-heat it, strain out the plant matter first. Heating the leaves and flowers again tends to alter the medicinal benefit of the herbs.

Another use for red raspberry tea is as a soothing remedy for **leg and foot cramps**. Sipping 2-3 cups of the warm tea every two hours can quickly bring about relief. To give your cramp a real run for the money, save the strained red raspberry leaves, lump them together to form a poultice and apply them *warm* to the specific part of the body that's giving you trouble. Keep the herbs as warm as possible and remove them once they get cool.

Sort of gives a person new respect for a plant that has mostly been known for jazzing up jams and jellies. Yeah, I can hardly wait for summer each year so I can once again partake of this multi-purpose bush.

But I'll still hate the prickly parts.

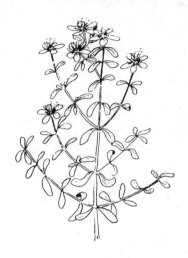

St. John's Wort—the Wound-Healing Herb with the Weird Name

Latin name: Hypericum perforatum
Medicinal parts: the entire plant
Forms: tea, extracted oil, tincture, extract
Marketing Rule #1: Always give your product an appealing name.

Marketing Rule #2: The word "wort" is usually not appealing.

I can hear it now. "I don't care if that herb is named after a Saint! I'm not boiling worts!"

First off, St. John's Wort has absolutely nothing to do with worts. It does, however, have plenty to do with **speeding the healing process when it comes to wounds, burns, bruises and painful neuralgia** and much more.

So, what's with the weird name? The plant, which buds around the time of the summer solstice (June 21), has pretty yellow flowers which contain tiny black dots. If you rub the petals and leaves between your fingers, a burnt purple oil which sort of resembles blood will ooze out. Early Christians who tried to connect normal occurrences in nature with religion, named the plant in honor of John the Baptist. They felt the plant actually grew from John the Baptist's blood after he was beheaded. They swore that on the anniversary of his death, August 29, the plant oozed its "bloody" oil in his memory. Kind of creepy, if you ask me. Nonetheless, the name stuck. And "Wort?" "Wort" is simply Old English for "plant."

No matter the strange name, this "Stephen King" herb with its oozing blood-red oil tendencies can do pretty amazing stuff. In plain talk, this herb is a keeper. Those little glands on the petals which spurt red contain a substance called *hypericin*. Hypericin is the activating ingredient that allows St. John's Wort to work it's herbal magic. Modern chemists have studied *hypericin* and discovered, to their surprise, that it contains **anti-viral, anti-depressive, anti-bacterial, anti-fungal and anti-inflammatory capabilities.**

That hypericin truly earns a spot in the big leagues when it comes to St. John's Wort's wound-healing abilities. When St. John's Wort oil or tincture is poured into wounds, the **wounds have a tendency to heal faster and reject infection.** The rejection to infection is thanks in part to the natural antibiotic chemicals hidden within that blood-red oil in the petals. In addition, the plant also has the ability to **reduce inflammation as well as lessen the pain from wounds** since it works directly on the nerves. However, St. John's Wort oil or tincture (which can be purchased as a topical homeopathic under the name "hypericum spray") tends to work *best* when used on fresh, dirty wounds (such as those where outside bacteria is also present). For "clean" wounds—i.e., when you cut yourself with a knife—calendula tincture, oil or ointment is a superior choice.

Never was the wort's wonders felt more truly than when a friend of mine took a tumble off of his mountain bike. He fell toward the gravel-strewn bike path with the palms of his hands skidding across the jagged rocks. Most of the scrapes were tiny surface cuts. However, there were two deep cuts near his right thumb that started throbbing with pain. My friend said there wasn't a lot of blood but the wounds stung like crazy. When he returned home, he washed off the surface dirt and gravel particles. Then he remembered that little bottle of hypericum spray he had in the medicine chest. After saturating both hands with the tincture, he noticed an almost immediate reduction in surface pain. Figuring the stuff was doing something worthwhile, he kept applying the tincture to his wounds about every hour as well as covering the cuts with a thick layer of calendula ointment. He said that after several hours, not only did the pain subside greatly, but he could actually see the wounds begin to heal. The following day, he used the tincture several times and by the third day, with the help of the calendula ointment he was scar-free one week after his bike dive. (See the chapter on calendula, page 15 for more info).

St. John's Wort oil can always be used in place or alternated with the tincture. The crimson oil is one of the most soothing, healing oils I've ever used. Unfortunately, sometimes the extracted oil is difficult to find in your local herb/health store.

Purists believe it is best to make your own, however, that isn't as easy as it sounds. Concocting the oil is not difficult—finding the *fresh* herb is. The stuff used to grow wild in every field and meadow. But in the last decade, it has been re-classified as a "noxious weed." Ranchers discovered that when their livestock ate the yellow flower, the animals often became ill and sometimes died. Thus, over the years, there was a concerted effort to destroy the plant. Apparently, enough people ripped this plant up by its root straps to make it darn near impossible to find in the wild. There's the occasional field here and there where you'll still see the herb weaving through the soil. But mostly, the only time you're going to see the plant is if you cultivate it from seed or seedling yourself. Once established in shady and moist soil, St. John's Wort can literally homestead your property, becoming a hearty perennial.

If you are able to locate the herb in the wild, here are some facts to consider. St. John's Wort often grows in clusters. However, the tiny seeds tend to blow no farther than 50 feet away. So, in the wild, when you find one grouping of plants, there should be another smaller or larger cluster within a 50 foot radius. Depending upon your geographical location, the flowers bloom anytime between the middle of June to the end of August. However, once they start blooming, they can be extremely short-lived. The Wort's blooming lifespan ranges anywhere from seven days to four weeks, depending upon the climate. (The moister and cooler it is the better). After its short-lived life, the delicate flowers quickly curl up and die. I have found that it is best to pick St. John's Wort flowers when there are both fresh flowers *and* buds on the plant. For some reason, the resulting extracted oil takes on a deeper red color and sweeter scent.

To make the healing oil, simply follow the directions on page 190 under the heading "Herbal Oil Extraction," using both the leaf and flower. However, *the base oil to use for St. John's Wort is olive oil because it has a better ability to pull the healing essence out of the plant.* Homemade oils should last up to two years if they are kept in a dark bottle and away from heat.

St. John's Wort oil is also an excellent treatment for **burns caused by the sun or caused by the stove**. However, there are two things to remember: *St. John's Wort should never be cooked on the stove. Use the slower method of placing the jar in the sun, Secondly, the oil must only be made in a base of flax seed oil so as not to aggravate the burn and cause blistering.* Not only can this oil work to dull the pain of the burn, it can also lower the temperature of the skin and speed the healing process when used quickly and continually. Some folks have found that when they add 3-5 drops of lavender pure essential oil to the St. John's Wort extracted oil, the burn heals even more quickly.

Because St. John's Wort soothes the nerves, relieves pain and reduces inflammation this amazing oil has been used in the treatment of **sciatica, arthritis, spinal problems, pain of the coccyx (the small triangular bone at the base of the spine) and neuralgia**. The best way to apply the extracted oil for such ailments is to gently heat five to ten tablespoons over low heat. DO NOT LET IT BOIL! Once the oil is warm, carefully soak either a cotton pad or clean cotton cloth in the liquid. BE CAREFUL! If the oil is too hot, you can get a serious burn! However, the oil does need to be warm when you place it over the afflicted area. You can tape the cotton pad to the area you want to treat or use the cotton pad to simply "paint" the oil on the skin. Gently massage the area until all the oil absorbs into the skin. As mentioned, a flax seed oil base is mandatory for burns. For pain problems that don't involve burns or scalds, olive oil is the one to choose. If you want to boost St. John's Wort's external pain relieving effects, add equal parts arnica oil. This blend is especially effective for low back pain and sciatica.

Often, folks who experience semi-regular bouts with pain also take the herb internally to sort of "boost up" its healing powers. This can be done in tea form, extract, tincture or in the homeopathic form of *hypericum* *6x* or *10x*. DO NOT TAKE THE OIL INTERNALLY! The normal dosage for tea is one teaspoon of the dried herb to 8 oz. of hot distilled water. For the extract and tincture, dissolve 10-15 drops in 4 oz. of warm distilled water. The dosage amount of the homeopathic *hypericum* depends greatly upon what painful ailment you are treating. It can range from two tablets every two hours to only two tablets a day for no longer than three weeks at a time. For this reason, it is always best to consult with a homeopathic doctor who can better gauge the amount you will need.

As a tea, St. John's Wort has been successful in some cases as an **anti-depressant in cases of deep psychological anxiety brought on by everything from grief and personal turmoil to hormonal imbalances during PMS or menopause which cause sadness, irritability or the inability to function on a daily basis.** Once again, that highly-regarded hypericin works to interfere with the chemical in the body called monoamine oxidase (MAO) which can contribute to depression. Chemical MAO inhibitors found in many anti-depressant drugs are much stronger than the natural MAO inhibitors within St. John's Wort. However, St. John's Wort has proven to work more gently on the body when taken regularly for a minimum 2-3 months. Studies in Europe have shown that over a three to six month test period, 2-3 cups of St. John's Wort tea a day had the ability to gradually bring those suffering from depression out of the blues. Feelings of "greater self worth," "more interest in life," and "normal sleep patterns," are just a few of the glowing reports attributed to St. John's Wort tea. Mind you, it's not an instant cure for chronic depression and it does not work on everyone. However, for those who are affected positively by it, the herb can be a godsend.

The herb also worked its uplifting magic in extract and tincture form when 10-20 drops were placed in 6 oz. of warm distilled water and drunk daily for two months at a time with one week off in between. **It is important to note that, as an anti-depressant, the tea/extract/tincture of St. John's Wort should be administered under a doctor's supervision.** Long term, continuous use of the herb (defined as over seven months) is not recommended for depression since too much of the plant could cause toxicity in some people. However, it is being used in many alternative circles to help wean people off the drug **Prozac**. This *does not* mean that if you are currently taking Prozac (or *any* other drug for depression) that you toss it in the trash and start chugging St. John's Wort. Never, never, *never* quit any anti-depressant drug cold-turkey. It is vital that you wean your body off of the drug slowly and always with the help of a doctor. With your doctor or holistic practitioner's permission, you can take small doses of St. John's Wort during that weaning process as it may make the process less shocking to the body.

Boy, this herb's amazing abilities don't stop there. For literally hundreds of years, St. John's Wort has been used to help kids who suffer from **chronic bed wetting**. As long as the problem is not rooted in the emotions, St. John's Wort may be able to help. The normal dose is 5-10 drops of the extract or tincture under the child's tongue, taken 1-2 hours before bedtime. Many herbalists stress the importance of paying close attention to the child's diet. White bread, white sugar, processed meats, soft drinks, caffeine-loaded beverages and chocolate should be eliminated from the diet since they stimulate the body as well as gradually break down its ability to properly nourish the system.

Recently, one of the most important studies in the use of St. John's Wort has been in the treatment of **AIDS**. However, I have to stress that the bulk herb itself is not being used—rather, a "standardized extract" which can only be prescribed by a doctor. The extract has also shown, in controlled studies, to be effective against the HIV virus. When the standardized extract was injected into mice which were infected with viruses that cause leukemia, the herb was found to have "totally prevented disease." In AIDS patients who are currently undergoing experimentation with St. John's Wort extract, patients have reported everything from "greater energy and weight gain" to "improved appetite and increased immune function." All of these studies are obviously only in the preliminary stages but at least science is attempting to bridge the gap with natural medicine.

There are always cautions and St. John's Wort is no exception. The hypericin—while healing—has been shown to cause photosensitivity in some people. This simply means that **if you have a sensitivity to sun—especially if you are fair-skinned—large doses of St. John's Wort used either**

internally or externally, can cause even greater sensitivity to the sun which can result in red skin and sometimes blisters. This does not happen to everyone with fair skin, but it's safe to say that if you wish to use St. John's Wort oil and you fall into that "sensitive" category, stay out of the sun and away from heat lamps! **In addition, it's best to stay off alcohol, coffee, chocolate, narcotics, diet pills, asthma inhalants, nasal decongestants and amphetamines because they can interfere with the action of the herb.**

Yes, this plant may have an odd name. But once you see what the "Wort" can do, you'll always want this "Saintly" herb near the front of the shelf.

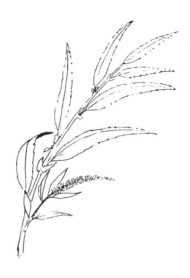

WHITE WILLOW—
BARKING UP THE
HEADACHE TREE

Latin name: *Salix alba*
Medicinal parts: bark
Forms: tea, extract, capsule

Once upon a time in a faraway land a long time ago, whenever people felt headaches, swollen joints or a fever coming on, they would walk into the woods (back then, everyone lived near or in the woods) and locate the white willow tree. Finding the tree, they would carefully break off some new branches. Upon returning to their cabin, they'd take a hunting knife and tear the bark off the smooth branches, revealing the orange-tinted pulp. They would crush the bark between their palms and then drop it into a cup or two of boiling water, letting it bubble for 20 minutes. They would then strain the bark from the liquid, drink the light brown tea, lie down and in about an hour or so, their **headache/fever/swollen joints** would feel much better.

This ritual into the woods went on for thousands of years. Then one day a group of chemists decided they wanted to find out what made this white willow bark so powerful. They took the white willow bark and examined it under a microscope and found the one component that reduced fevers, stopped headaches and relieved swollen joints. And one French chemist decided to call it "salicine." All the scientists were thrilled and rejoiced in the fact that they, with their infinite wisdom, could actually *improve* on nature.

And so these chemists took that one little component of the white willow bark, synthesized it, turned it into acetylsalicylic acid, made it into a round, white pill, stuck it in a bottle and made a fortune. And what did they call this little white synthetic pill?

Aspirin—The most widely used drug in the world today.

Now, some of you might be saying that science did us all a favor by discovering the active component in the bark of that white willow tree. But like all synthetic drugs that have been pulled, poked and pricked from a whole plant, root or bark, you don't get the full, *balanced* benefit of the natural herb.

For example, many people who take aspirin on a regular basis complain of stomach upset and irritation. Some heavy-duty aspirin users worry that stomach ulcers are a high price to pay for headache relief.

These symptoms are non-existent with the whole herb: white willow bark. Why? Because the bark contains the balancing agents that offset stomach irritation, ulcers and the like. When those clever chemists isolated the one section of the bark that was responsible for headache relief—mainly the part containing the "salicine" or "salicin," as we now call it—they threw away the herb's equalizing parts that make the whole herb work effectively and without the irritating side effects. Those "other parts" that the chemists tossed aside so that they could "improve on nature" include tannins which are actually great for digestion.

While some herbalists admit that white willow bark may not offer the same quick results as aspirin sometimes does, (depending upon the individual, it may take more of the white willow bark to have the same effect as aspirin), it is generally agreed that white willow bark is easier on the system than aspirin as well as a dependable pain-relieving herbal remedy.

And scientists even have to agree that white willow bark basically does the same thing as its chemical counterpart. It just does it in a different way. To explain: today's aspirin was created by chemically altering the naturally-occurring salicin into salicylic acid. (Later, salicylic acid was further altered to create acetylsalicylic acid which is what modern day aspirin is based upon). What is worth mentioning though, is that when you ingest white willow bark tea, your body *naturally* converts the bark's salicin into salicylic acid. Further, because of this natural phenomenon, science has discovered that the salicin is then able to work more effectively— often times enabling the body to take better advantage of the herb's pain-relieving ability. What this means in a nutshell is what herbalists have been hammering on: when you isolate an active ingredient in a plant and throw out everything else, you miss out on the total healing effect. What I like to say is "Use the whole plant if you want to treat the whole person." Period.

First and foremost, think of white willow bark whenever you need a **natural pain killer**. Throughout history, white willow bark was always associated with what was called "hot" conditions or ailments. "Hot" conditions would fall into the category of fevers, neuralgia and swollen joints. White willow bark won't knock you out like some pain killers can and it may not work for serious, chronic discomfort. However, it's definitely worth a try.

Since aspirin is used daily by those suffering from arthritis or **rheumatic conditions**, let's start with these first. Because white willow bark is chock-full of salicylates (**natural anti-inflammatory** components which help to take the heat out of "hot" joints), the herb can be a nature-friendly alternative to aspirin. One could take white willow in tea form at 3-4 cups each day for three weeks with one week off. The sweet and "musty" white willow bark tea is made by combining one heaping teaspoon of the bark with 10 oz of distilled water, bringing it to a full rolling boil for five minutes, letting it steep covered for 20 minutes, straining and then drinking. Besides being one of the least expensive herbs on the market, white willow bark is also the most economical. You can re-use the initial teaspoon of bark up to three times without losing a lot of the pain killing action.

The tea works very effectively to **reduce fevers** as well as the **aches and pains of colds and flu**. I have used white willow bark many times when I had a cold and it has always worked like a trooper. For the first one or two days of the cold or flu, you can take up to four cups of the tea or three to four of the capsules each day.

Personally, I don't think the capsules work half as effectively as the tea since it can sometimes take them hours to burst open and start working. However, if that's the only way you like to take your herbs and you want to get this one inside your body, then by all means take the capsule.

Because the tea tends to soothe as well as cool hot, irritated and painful conditions, it has been used as a stop-gap remedy for **bladder infections** and **gastric inflammations**. Those who have used the tea for bladder complaints say that it reduces the inflammation in the urethra and makes urination less painful. For gastric inflammation, the tea works best when combined with a teaspoon of plantain. (See page 123 for more info on plantain). Mind you, if either of these conditions are chronic, the tea will only mildly placate the problem. As always, if the problem worsens or does not improve within 36 hours, see a doctor immediately.

For the nature-lover, foraging for fresh white willow bark can be a somewhat fulfilling experience. That is, if you're into outdoor activities with an excitement quotient of negative two. First off, it is very important that you make sure you can positively identify the white willow tree. If you are the least bit unsure if the tree in question is indeed the mighty willow, forego home collecting and head down to your herb/health store to purchase the herb.

If you are certain you've found the white willow tree, hunt for the branches that appear the newest. These would be identified usually by a smoother bark which is easily peeled with the use of only your fingers. The older branches are okay but they are harder to harvest and tend to have less of the medicinal value. When you find a good branch, snap it off and gently pull back the fresh bark to reveal the light orange colored pulp. If there is any moisture in the tree, you should be able to smell the slightly sweet, musty aroma that explicitly spells w-i-l-l-o-w. Once you have stripped the bark from the stem, tear it into smaller sections and allow it to dry outside in indirect sunlight. Once the bark becomes brittle, you can then make a tea.

As long as we're out in the woods, it's worth mentioning that if you love the outdoors and camping, white willow bark can work as a wonderful first aid tree when you're in a pinch. For instance, the fresh stripped bark—crushed, moistened with water and made into a loose poultice—makes a good pack for **bleeding wounds**.

Thanks to the bark's high tannin content, it has strong astringent properties as well as pretty decent antiseptic capabilities.

Another use for the bark—in and out of the woods—is as a strong but gentle skin wash for **skin ulcers, eczema** or **infected wounds**. To make the wash, simply add two cups of the bark to four cups of boiling water. Allow the mixture to simmer for at least half an hour. I usually don't strain out the bark because I think the longer it's in the pot, the stronger the solution will be. The other advantage is that you can always scoop the bark out of the pot and pack it around the skin condition for added medicinal value. This herbal skin wash can be used externally as often as needed. If you want to give the wash an energetic boost, add a tablespoon of boric acid to the liquid after the mixture has been allowed to simmer.

The powdered bark also works well for **minor burns**. Just crush the bark with a mortar and pestle, add enough water to make a paste and you've got a very soothing poultice that can cool the heat from surface burns.

Externally, white willow bark tea is used as a hair rinse for those folks suffering from **dandruff**. If used regularly (two to three times a week) you could see a gradual reduction in the dandruff problem. On the hair front, there are theories that the same rinse (and internal use of the tea) may help prevent and/or reduce the chance of **baldness** in both men and women.

Even though this herb is soothing to the body, there are cautions. **Just as pregnant women are advised to not take aspirin because of possible birth defects, the same applies for white willow bark.** Obviously the herb is not as strong or intrusive as aspirin. But because aspirin's a kissing cousin to the bark, the caution marker goes up.

There's yet another aspirin connection caution. **Children under 16 with colds, flu or chicken pox are told by doctors not to take aspirin because of the risk of developing Reye's Syndrome—a potentially fatal condition. The same is true for white willow bark.** Now, there has never been a documented case of anyone under 16 with the above mentioned ailments contracting Reye's Syndrome. But it's better to be safe than sorry.

Can you overdose on white willow bark tea? I've never heard of anyone doing that. However, **long-term use of the herb in**

any of its forms has tended to act a as sex depressant. Being the "Queen of Moderation," I would cap my bark consumption at four cups a day when colds and flu hit and a limit of 2-3 cups each day when the tea is taken for pain or inflammation.

About 8-12 hours after drinking white willow bark tea, you may experience a slight purging from the bowels. White willow is not indicated for constipation in any herbal reference guide I can find. But over the years, I have known the herb to work overtime in that department.

Not too shabby for a common bark that grows prolifically across the country.

But perhaps we shouldn't talk too loudly about the extra benefits of the white willow bark.

Some bored chemist out there might get ideas.

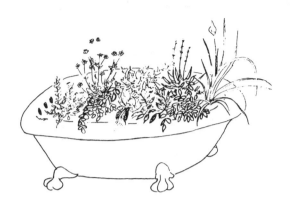

THE HERBAL BATH HATH WHAT IT TAKES!

One soak in an herbal bath and you may never go back to the normal routine. Plain water is okay, but add an herb or pure essential oil and you've got a bath with extra "umph" that'll bring relief to whatever ails you.

It's very important to remember that while herbal baths can be invigorating, rejuvenating and relaxing, their main objective is to act as an external aid for better health. Herbal baths work two ways: First, the water helps pull waste and debris locked deep within the tissues and pores of the skin. Secondly, a mere 20 minute soak in an herbal bath can rev up your circulation. Better circulation means the blood is moving rapidly through your veins and bringing life to sluggish limbs.

Because herbal baths are supposed to be geared toward helping you physically, you approach them differently than you would the normal "soap & water" affair. So, **the first rule when taking an herbal bath is do not use soap or any other bath salts, beads or bubbles**. Not only do these have chemicals in them, they diminish or dilute the effects of the medicinal herbs. If you want to wash your skin before taking your herb bath, by all means take a quick shower and then head for the herbs.

Temperature is an important factor. Get the water too hot and you may end up prostrate on the bathroom floor. Get it too tepid and the herbs or oils won't have enough heat to activate their "juices." I have found the best temperature for an herbal bath is between 100°-101°F. If you are feeling on the weak side due to an illness, fatigue or physical pain, keep the temperature around 95°-99°F so the heat doesn't pull the remaining strength out of you. There are many old herbal books from around the world that insist the hotter the bath, the "quicker the cure." I suppose this makes some sense. The idea being that the faster I can get the junk out of my pores, the faster I'll be back on my feet. The only problem is the hotter the bath, the more it depletes your body of water. For those folks who are already not feeling fit as a fiddle, a fiery hot bath could take a lot out of you, causing dizziness, shaking, headaches, rapid heartbeat and dehydration. This eradicates the reason for taking the bath in the first place. So, take my advice and keep the herbal bath at a reasonable temperature.

While you are in the herb bath, **it is always a good idea to have a large glass of room temperature water in arm's reach to sip on at five minute intervals**. This can help equalize the body temperature if it gets too hot as well as replenish the body with fluids lost when the hot water drains the pores. In addition, **I strongly recommend that you drink 8-10 oz. of room temperature water after you get out of the bath and dry off**. After only 20 minutes, your body will be dehydrated and will crave water to replenish what was lost via the pores.

Another important point is to keep the bathroom temperature around 70°-75°F and *make sure there are no drafts*. The last thing you need is to get a chill.

There are four ways to use herbs in a bath: tea, extracted oil, pure essential oil and dried herbs packed into a muslin sack. For times that you really want to perk up the bath, you can use both the tea and one of the oil forms together, although it can sometimes be too harsh on sensitive skin. Here are the four forms explained in more detail.

Tea bath—Consider this like soaking in one big ol' cup o' tea. The usual ratio is three cups of the dried herb to five quarts of tap water. Heat the water in a large pot that can accommodate the liquid (such as a deep pasta pot) or divide the herbs and water equally into two separate pots. Allow the water to almost come to a boil and then turn off the burner. Immediately add the dried herbs, mixing them with a wooden spoon so that they soak into the water. Cover and let the mixture steep for 20-30 minutes and then strain out the herbs. Add the liquid to a hot bath and soak for 25-40 minutes. Do not re-heat the herbal mixture because the active ingredients within the plant's volatile oils will be leeched out.

Oil extraction—This is just like your typical bath oil except, of course, for its medicinal benefit. (To see how to make your own herbal oil extraction, turn to page 190). You can add as much as four tablespoons of the extracted oil to the bath water. Be careful when getting in and out of the tub since the combination of oil and porcelain can equal a slippery surface. Also, depending upon what base oil you use for the extraction, your skin will absorb some of it but there will also be a layer left on the skin after getting out of the tub. If your skin has a tendency to be oily and you don't want to add to it, choose apricot kernel oil as the base oil since it absorbs more quickly and is much lighter in texture to the touch.

Pure essential oils—These are oils which have been steam distilled from the flower or plant. To make sure you are buying an essential oil and not an extracted oil, the bottle *must* say the words "pure essential oil," "steam-distilled essential oil" or simply "essential oil." Essential oils are extremely concentrated—which means a little goes a long way. Their measurement is in drops *not* spoonfuls. Too much of an essential oil dose can cause skin irritation, itching and sometimes rashes so always keep to the recommended drop dose. It's always best to draw your bath, undress, stand in the water with your little bottle of essential oil and drop the aromatic liquid into the bath right before you plunge in. Dropping the oil in while the bath is running tends to evaporate the essence and you lose most of the healing benefit. To extend the aromatic essence, try placing 10 drops of the essential oil into a tablespoon of either apricot kernel oil or whole milk and then swish the mixture into the bath water before you get into the tub. There are water soluble essential oils on the market these days that have a longer-lasting effect since they blend with the water and don't evaporate as quickly. If you can't find water soluble essential oils, you can combine the regular pure essential oil with something called "Red Turkey Oil." (No, not *Wild Turkey* and no, it's *not* made from turkeys.) After adding 8-10 drops of the pure essential oil, place one teaspoon of Red Turkey Oil in the water. This will help disperse the essential oil more evenly and allow it to last longer before it finally evaporates.

Muslin sack—This has the same purpose as the tea bath, except the effect is milder. Buy or make a muslin bag approximately 4" x 6" square and secure with a string tie to close. Stuff it full of the herb or combination of herbs that you want. Draw your bath and put the herb-filled bag into the water, squeezing it often to release the herbal essence. You can keep the bag in the water while you soak, occasionally gently rubbing the muslin against your skin to receive a more concentrated herbal benefit. If you wring it out and let it air dry, the bag should last you for 2-3 baths.

The herbal baths that follow have the ability to do their job naturally and effectively. If you experience any skin irritations or unpleasant effects, discontinue the bath.

Here's to a happy herbal bath experience!

Cayenne bath:

The effect: To *really, really* warm up the body and increase circulation.

How to make it: Tea bath or muslin sack. *However, use only 2-3 tablespoons of the dry powdered herb* in the water or muslin sack. The heat generated from this bath can be *very* uncomfortable if too much of the powdered herb is used.

When to use it: Morning, noon or evening. Cayenne won't keep you awake but it will keep your body *very* warm or hot for up to four hours.

How long a soak: 20 minutes tops! If you start to feel uncomfortable or your skin begins to burn, get out immediately!

How many times per week: Two to three. However, never overdo it because too much use of this bath can irritate sensitive skin.

Chamomile bath:

The effect: To calm and soothe frazzled nerves. Soothes skin rashes—especially eczema.

How to make it: Tea bath or muslin sack. The pure essential oil is too expensive to use.

When to use it: Best in the evening since it tends to relax the nerves.

How long a soak: 30-40 minutes.

How many times per week: Three to four.

Comfrey bath:

The effect: To soothe skin inflammation, burns, bruises, rheumatism or whenever there is any ligament, tissue or bone-related problem. Also, a wonderful, natural skin softener.

How to make it: Tea bath or muslin sack. Use either the *fresh* leaves or the *dried root powder.*

When to use it: Whenever you need relief from ailments mentioned under "effect."

How long a soak: 30-40 minutes.

How many times per week: Three to four.

Eucalyptus bath:

The effect: To open up clogged sinuses, relieve chest congestion and ease muscle stiffness.

How to make it: Pure essential oil. Only 8-10 drops maximum.

When to use it: Morning or afternoon. Evening can be too stimulating. However, if you are suffering from congestion, by all means, take a soak after sunset.

How long a soak: 20-25 minutes.

How many times per week: One to three.

Ginger bath:

The effect: To ease sore muscles, back pain, shake off a cold during the first stages and to jump-start circulation.

How to make it: Tea bath or muslin sack. *However, use only 3-5 tablespoons of the powdered root in the tea water or muslin sack.* One cup of table salt or Epsom salts can be added to give the bath a bit more punch.

When to use it: In the evening. Ginger tends to increase perspiration. Because of this, it is not a good idea to take a ginger bath and then go outside since you may get a chill and risk further muscular cramping or pain.

How long a soak: 15-20 minutes *tops*/20 minutes maximum if you add the salt.

How many times per week: Two to three.

Lavender bath:

The effect: To relax body and mind, soothe the senses and promote sleep.

How to make it: Tea bath, muslin sack or 10-15 drops of lavender pure essential oil or lavender extracted oil. Combining the oil with the tea bath really revs up the herbal effects!

When to use it: Usually in the evening since you will want to drift off to sleep when you get out of the tub. However, try the bath anytime you need to relax.

How long a soak: 30-40 minutes.

How many times per week: Three to five.

Mustard bath:

The effect: To warm your body and relieve chest congestion. This bath can also ease muscular pain.

How to make it: Tea bath or muslin sack. *However, use only 1/2—1 cup of the dried, powdered herb.*

When to use it: Only in the evening or when you are sure you won't be venturing outside the house. Mustard powder is *extremely* strong and produces lots of perspiration. It is very important to stay warm after getting out of a mustard bath.

How long a soak: 30-40 minutes.

How many times per week: Three to four.

Peppermint bath:

The effect: To cool the body, stimulate the senses and clear the sinuses.

How to make it: Tea bath, muslin sack or 10-15 drops of the pure essential oil or peppermint extracted oil. Combining the pure essential oil or extracted oil with the tea will be even more stimulating.

When to use it: A morning or afternoon bath. Works well in the summertime when you need a cool lift. Also a good bath for itching skin due to poison ivy or skin rashes.

How long a soak: 30-40 minutes.

How many times per week: Three to five.

Rosemary bath:

The effect: To give your body a wonderful energy boost, clear the mind and help you to concentrate.

How to make it: Tea bath, muslin sack or 10-15 drops of the pure essential oil or rosemary extracted oil. Combining the pure essential oil or the extracted oil with the tea will really stimulate the senses.

When to use it: Great morning "wake-up!" bath or afternoon picker-upper. The bath can sometimes be too stimulating for the evening.

How long a soak: 20-30 minutes.

How many times per week: Three to five.

Thyme bath:

The effect: For nervous over stimulation, depression, muscular weakness due to injury, rheumatism and sprains.

How to make it: Tea bath or 10-15 drops of the pure essential oil or thyme extracted oil. I don't recommend combining the tea with the oils since it can be too strong.

When to use it: In the evening since the bath has a tendency to calm and soothe the nervous system. It is best to take thyme bath and then relax with soft music or go to sleep.

How long a soak: 20-30 minutes.

How many times per week: Two to three. If nervousness or depression become a chronic condition, it might be a good idea to get a doctor's opinion.

Aching-Overworked bath blend:

The effect: Helps relieve aching muscles, soothe bruises and loosen stiff joints.

How to make it: Tea bath or muslin sack. Combine equal amounts of comfrey root powder, ginger root powder and arnica flowers. Because you are working with more than one herb, you can cut the tea bath recipe in half (i.e., 1 1/2 cups of the combined herbs to 2 1/2 cups of tap water.

When to use it: Works best in the evening when you can kick back and relax in bed afterwards.

How long a soak: 20-25 minutes. If the ginger starts to burn, get out of the bath and reduce the amount of ginger in the blend the next time.

How many times per week: Two to three.

Meditation bath blend:

The effect: Helps one to become more "centered," easing the transition into a calm, meditative state.

How to make it: Tea bath or muslin sack. Combine equal amounts of cloves, cedarwood chips, sandalwood, garden sage and myrrh powder. *Because these herbs are very potent, the tea needs only to be made with one cup of the **combined** herbs to three quarts of tap water.* For the muslin sack, make sure all the herbs are mixed together so none get left out of the sack.

When to use it: Whenever you want to relax and think lovely thoughts.

How long a soak: 20-25 minutes. If your skin feels "prickly" or starts to burn, get out of the bath and discontinue use of this potent blend.

How many times per week: One to two. More than that and your skin may get irritated.

All of these herb baths work great for adults. If the kids want to get into the act, you'll need to **reduce the proportions by one half to one quarter the original amounts. This is especially true for youngsters under the age of 12 and for** *any* **child with fair or sensitive skin.**

Extra care must be taken with babies to make sure their delicate skin is not harmed by the herbs and particularly the pure essential oils. While both chamomile and lavender pure essential oils are meant to calm and soothe, chamomile can be far too strong when used on a baby's tender skin. However, one drop (and I mean *one drop*) of lavender pure essential oil in a baby's bath water has done wonders to quiet and calm the most cranky of newborns.

Yes, the simple art of the bath can take on new dimensions when a favorite flower, leaf, root or oil is added to the water. I warn you though, this stuff is habit forming.

Bathing may never be the same again.

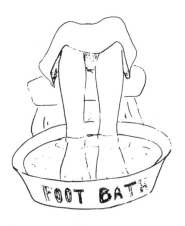

FOOT BATH

PUTTING YOUR FOOT IN THE RIGHT CONCOCTION

For a moment, look on the soles of the feet as if they were a couple of porous sponges, absorbing whatever is soaked into them. The blood stream then takes over and chugs the substance all through your body and before you know it, you just might be tasting it or seeing that substance in another form.

Don't believe it? Experiments were conducted where crushed garlic dipped in olive oil was spread on the soles of the feet. The feet were wrapped in plastic wrap and the garlic held in place for two hours. Within the two hour period, participants in this odd study swore they tasted raw garlic in their mouth.

Warm castor oil was used in another treatment. The feet were covered with a thick coating of the stuff and massaged until the castor oil was fully absorbed into the soles. The following day, those folks with the slippery feet noticed that their urine had strange little pools of oil floating in it. Needless to say, naysayers were convinced.

Yes, the feet are powerful appendages, pulsating and propelling liquid nutrients throughout the body. Some old herbal books insist that there's nothing like a good ol' fashioned foot bath to relieve **pain in the lower back, pelvic discomfort, menstrual and**

stomach cramps and even prostate congestion. What a hot foot bath does is warm the body quickly, producing a sweat and discharging trapped congestion from organs and joints.

It is important to remember when trying a foot bath to keep the body warm since excessive perspiration can result in a chill. I've found that if you bundle up in a heavy blanket, keeping only your calves and head exposed, you can get results quickly. It's always good to have a cool (not ice cold!) washcloth nearby to lay across your forehead and/or nape of neck to take the edge off the heat and wipe away the sweat.

A plain hot water foot bath is one of the oldest ways used to break a fever, relieve congestion and quickly warm the body. I know that after 15 minutes, I feel more relaxed, less sore and begin to generate much more circulation throughout my body. After 30 minutes—the maximum time spent in a foot bath—I'm ready to face the world anew ... after a quick nap, of course.

Plain water foot baths are good and have done wonders throughout the ages. But I do prefer perking up the water with a little herbal boost.

You can turn to the chapter "Herbal Baths" (page 146) and use any of those herbal concoctions for your foot bath. However, the herb to basin o' water ratio for a foot bath would be *no more than one half cup of the **dried** herb or three to five drops of any of the pure essential oils or extracted oils* to one average size bucket of water. For example, just as peppermint works in the bath to cool and revitalize, the dried herb, pure essential oil or extracted oil have the same effect on the feet—with the added benefit of relieving hot, swollen or aching feet.

The water should hover somewhere between 99-103° F.—never higher. After the 30 minute maximum foot soak, rinse your feet off with lukewarm water to gently bring down the body's temperature. If you have perspired profusely, take a quick dip in the shower to rinse your body. Most importantly, stay warm.

The cautions for the foot baths are important to keep in mind. *Do not under any circumstance attempt any kind of foot bath if you have diabetes, chronic circulation problems, hardening of the arteries or frostbite.* **If you are menstruating heavily, the foot bath may aggravate the condition. In a case like that, make sure the water is** only **100** degrees and soak your feet for only **15 minutes**.

In addition to the baths described in the "Herbal Bath" chapter, here are seven soaks designed for the feet.

Cayenne & Ginger foot bath:

The effect: To *really* warm the body and whip the circulation into gear!

How to make it: Three tablespoons of ginger root powder and one tablespoon of dried cayenne powder to one basin of hot tap water.

When to use it: Anytime you want to warm your body. Great for those wintry nights.

How long a soak: 20-25 minutes. If your feet start to burn or there is any discomfort, take your feet out of the foot bath. *It is normal for your feet to feel very hot for one to four hours after a cayenne/ginger foot bath.*

How many times per week: Two to three.

Coltsfoot foot bath:

The effect: To reduce swollen feet.

How to make it: One to two cups of the fresh or dried herb to one basin of hot tap water

When to use it: In the evening when you can relax and put your feet up afterwards.

How long a soak: 20 minutes.

How many times per week: Three to five.

Epsom salt foot bath:

The effect: To relieve soreness, throbbing and inflammation.

How to make it: One half to one cup of Epsom salt.

When to use it: Morning, afternoon or evening—whenever you need relief.

How long a soak: 20-30 minutes.

How many times per week: Two to three.

Horsetail foot bath:

The effect: To help reduce and even eliminate the "sweaty feet" syndrome. May also strengthen thin or split toenails due to the herb's high silicon and selenium content. Can soothe cracked skin and inflammation of the nail bed.

How to make it: Soak 4 oz. of horsetail in cold water for 12 hours. Then, heat the mixture gently but *do not* let it boil. Pour contents directly into the foot bath.

When to use it: Whenever you need the benefits it provides.

How long a soak: 20 minutes.

How many times per week: Every night if necessary.

Parsley foot bath:

The effect: To relieve painful menstrual cramping and menopausal discomfort.

How to make it: Three to four cups of the whole fresh plant to one basin of hot tap water.

When to use it: Anytime you need relief from the above-mentioned problems.

How long a soak: 30-45 minutes.

How many times per week: Four to six.

Tea tree oil foot bath:

The effect: One of the *best* all-natural, anti-fungal, anti-bacterial, antiseptic pure essential oils in the world. Used in a foot bath to kill athlete's foot, relieve joint stiffness and toenail infections—especially where a fungus is present.

How to make it: As with *all* pure essential oils, place tea tree oil in the water right before you soak your feet. Use 10-12 drops. For tough athlete's foot problems or nail infections, follow-up with five drops of the pure essential oil rubbed into the foot or directly over the nail.

When to use it: Whenever you need relief.

How long a soak: 30 minutes.

How many times per week: Three to five.

White willow bark foot bath:

The effect: To help eliminate sweaty feet.

How to make it: Boil one to two cups of the dried "cut" herb (i.e., not powdered) six cups of tap water. Simmer for 20 minutes then add the entire mixture to one basin of warm tap water. Allow mixture to cool down to a comfortable temperature before soaking your feet.

When to use it: Whenever you need relief.

How long a soak: 30-35 minutes.

How many times per week: Three to five.

A herbal foot bath might be just what you need to take a step in the right direction!

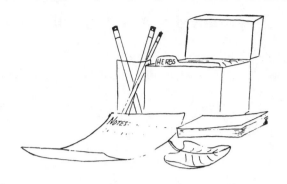

15 REALLY GOOD QUESTIONS PEOPLE ASK ABOUT HERBS

1. If medicinal herbs are so great, why is it more people don't use them?

I've found that many people look on herbs, in general, as harmless little plants, weeds and flowers with absolutely no connection to the healing field. Modern man has been indoctrinated during the 20th Century to trust high-tech chemical medicine over what many people refer to as "folk" or "backwoods" medicine. The irony is that numerous fast-acting drugs used today were created from a plant. A good example is aspirin which comes from a combination of white willow bark and meadowsweet or digitalis which is derived from the foxglove plant. However, awareness is shifting as many folks are tiring of prescription drugs and are looking for alternatives which are less toxic on the body. I feel that once herbs are given more serious consideration by health researchers and even doctors, their use won't be considered abnormal or even "alternative" in the future.

2. Are there any herbs I can take on a daily basis, indefinitely?

Personally, I hate crutches of any kind. I like to think that if one has a balanced nutritional diet, daily moderate exercise and a healthy outlook on life, the body should respond in kind. However, because of stress, pollution, frenzied lifestyles and poor diets, it is very easy to throw your body out of balance. For this reason, vitamins, minerals and herbs can be a beneficial addition to your life. However, I don't think anyone should take most herbs every single day of their life—no more than I think one should take the same vitamins every day for the rest of their life. If the body becomes saturated with one particular herb (or herbal formula), it could reject the plant and allergies might develop. Another possibility is the body could become immune to the benefits of the herb and then when you really need it, it ceases to work for you. There are, of course, exceptions to this rule. Some herbs, such as hawthorn berry and pau d' arco (two I did not cover in this book) have been taken on a daily basis for years at a time for specific health reasons. However, on average, one should moderate their use of most herbs. After all, the body is the engine—the herb is simply the fuel to get it moving in the right direction. For non-chronic problems, unless otherwise specified, my rule of thumb is to take an herb for 10-21 days with 7-10 days off in between.

3. Does it really matter how I take an herb?

This can depend upon what herb you are taking. Some herbs— such as echinacea—work best in tincture form. Other herbs—such as garlic—retain their highest potency in raw form. But in the real world, people often have very strong likes and dislikes. To some, the idea of eating a raw clove of garlic is unappetizing. Others may be turned off by the taste of an herb in tea or tincture form but don't mind it in capsule form. In fact, when capsules are an option, most people opt for them. The only problem with capsules is that if the gelatin capsule is not processed correctly, it may not break down in the stomach and release the herbs. There have been cases where people kept swallowing gelatin capsules and found no relief from the herb only to discover that the capsule was passing through their body whole and intact. For this reason, I'm not a big fan of capsules. Teas, tinctures and extracts move into the blood stream almost immediately to start their healing action. However, if it's between taking the herb the way you like it or not taking it at all, I'd say go with the way you like it.

4. Can I take herbs along with antibiotics?

Yes. In fact, many people who start taking herbs as an alternative after spending their life using antibiotics do just this. It's actually a good idea to wean yourself off the use of antibiotics, prescription drugs and over-the-counter drugs slowly—especially if your body has been used to taking chemical preparations for longer than two years. If you were to stop "cold turkey" and commence with herbs, your body may not know how to respond since it has been used to receiving synthetic drugs vs. natural substances. What I usually suggest people do when they've been taking chemical drugs is start out by introducing herbs into your body on a 70/30 scale. In other words, 70% chemical and 30% herbs. The next time, figure 60/40, then 50/50 and so on until herbs become the dominant treatment you choose. Mind you, the first time you combine the two, don't expect to see fast-acting results. Most natural substances are going to have to fight hard against their synthetic counterparts.

5. How long can I take herbs on my own before seeking a doctor's opinion?

The answer clearly depends upon what ailments you are treating and how serious the conditions. Self-medication is not always wise if you do not know what you are doing. This is especially true when it comes to herbs. If you decide to use herbal therapy, I strongly suggest that you not only read this book carefully but others as well to get as much information as you can about a specific herb or group of herbs. (For more books on herbs, see the bibliography on page 194). The answer I usually give people who ask this question is, if your symptoms continue for longer than four days, discontinue use of the herb and see a doctor. If the ailment you are attempting to treat is serious (such as pneumonia, food poisoning, blood poisoning or any deep-seated infection), my advice is always to seek a doctor's opinion first and then combine both herbal and drug therapy. Remember, it's not so much that the herbs fail to "take care of the problem," rather, it's the person using the herbs who might incorrectly diagnose the ailment and use the wrong herb. It is for this reason that continued education is vital.

6. Are recommended herbal doses the same for everyone (i.e., children, adults, the elderly)?

No. First of all, recommended doses are just that—recommended. Every adult body is different and the amount that works for one person may not be enough for another. In herbal medicine it is often a good idea to start off with one half to one third the suggested dose and then increase the dose if needed. However, there are special doses for children and the elderly. For children, you would use "Clark's Rule" to figure the appropriate dosage. Clark's Rule bases the herbal dose upon the child's weight. According to Clark's Rule, an "adult" is considered 150 pounds. Thus, all factoring is based upon 150 pounds. The child's weight is then divided into 150 to determine what approximate fraction of the "adult" dose to give. For example, if the child weighs 50 pounds, the fraction would be 50/150 or 1/3 the recommended adult dose. If the child weighs 30 pounds, the fraction would be 30/150 or 1/5 the recommended adult dose. If the child is at an in-between weight, always factor down rather than up to make sure you don't give the child too much of a dose.

When using extracts or tinctures, figure out the dose for a child by dividing the child's weight in half. That number is how many drops you need to administer (i.e., a 60 pound child would require 30 drops of the tincture or extract for each dose).

Children under the age of two years old, however, require extra-special care. Many herbs are considered too strong for their delicate bodies. However, an herb such as catnip (see page 24) which helps colic and high fever in infants is an appropriate remedy. Any mother who wishes to use herbal medicine should read as much as possible about herbal care directed specifically for children.

For the elderly—which is defined as anyone above the age of 65—the idea is not so much to limit the dose but to weaken the herbal preparation. So, if the recommend adult dose calls for one teaspoon of the dried herb to 8 oz. of hot distilled water, increase the water by one third, making it 12 oz. To further weaken the brew, limit the steeping or boiling time by one-half as well as increasing the amount of water.

External herbal preparations, however, do not need to be altered for either a child or an elderly person.

7. Is it wise to treat children's ailments such as ear infections, colic and colds with only herbs and no antibiotics?

Once again, you have to know exactly what you are doing or you must be working with a doctor. If you want to follow the "natural path," I feel it's best to have the support and experience of a trained holistic professional who knows your child and knows what will work most effectively. If the childhood ailment is detected early and treated with natural therapies, you can often avoid any serious repercussions. Also, the importance of the infant's or child's diet cannot be stressed enough. A balanced diet, complete with nutritious and unprocessed foods is a must for the child's health. Many childhood ailments can be caused by an unhealthy diet. For example, excessive milk products build up and create sinus congestion which can lead to respiratory difficulties. Too many sugar-filled foods leech the child's body of the nutritional building blocks which, in turn, break down the immune system. However, if the child does get sick and, after visiting the doctor and using natural remedies the child does not get better, then an antibiotic should be considered.

8. Can I take herbs, eat junk food and get the same results?

I'm afraid not. It's kind of like taking your car to get regular oil changes and tune-ups but filling the gas tank with dirty gasoline. After awhile, that bad fuel is going to work its way around the engine and create major problems. The same thing applies when you put non-nutritious food in your body with the occasional buffers of herbs to offset any "damage." No body can operate on "cheap fuel" since that "fuel" is what is pumping your heart and supporting your organs, tissues and muscles with the nourishment needed to keep going. To use herbs (or any form of natural therapy) as some kind of "magic bullet" to compensate for poor eating habits is not going to cut it.

9. Can herbs really help chronic conditions such as arthritis, heart disease and diabetes?

Yes. However, once again, diet is also very important. Once a balanced, nutritious diet becomes part of your lifestyle, herbs can be used to tone the organs, detoxify the system and support the body's natural ability to fight off whatever is causing the physical problem. Amazingly enough, there are thousands of cases where chronic conditions such as arthritis, heart disease and diabetes were reduced in severity by simply changing the diet and cutting out certain foods and beverages that were found to contribute to the specific problem. Once that was accomplished, herbs acted more as preventative care and support than as the "cure."

10. Why do I sometimes feel worse after taking an herb than better?

This is commonly referred to in herbal medicine as "The Law of Cure." This often happens to people whose bodies are overly toxic. When this is the case, the herbs have to work through the sludge first before they can do their job. As the herbs do this, the toxins are released—sometimes quickly through bowel elimination or excessive perspiration. Instead of starting to feel better, one can feel even worse. However, be assured that it is the result of your body doing its best to rid itself of the poisons and fight the infection. It is for this reason that I always suggest that one start with a lower amount of the recommended dose to see how the body reacts. Remember that in herbal medicine, more does not equal better!

11. How long can herbs last in their various forms before going bad or losing their potency?

The rule of thumb is as follows:

Fresh herbs: Fresh herbs should be used as soon as possible. I always like to have the herb go from the dirt to the pot within 30 minutes to retain the full fresh value.

Dried herbs: Dried herbs need to be kept in airtight, glass canisters in a dark, cool, dry spot. Depending upon the herb and what part of the plant is being stored (i.e., flowers, leaves, roots, bark, etc.), dried herbs can last from six months to one year before losing a portion of their potency. For this reason, unless you plan on using a whole lot of dried herbs, I would suggest only buying enough to last three to six months. Another tip: although powdered herbs are sometimes preferred over the more bulky "cut and sifted" variety, the powdered form tends to have less of a shelf life as far as the potency of the herb is concerned.

Capsules: Usually there is an expiration date on the bottle. However, if there is not, I try to use them within 12 months.

Tinctures & Extracts: Depending upon the solvent that is used (alcohol, glycerin, vinegar or water), tinctures and extracts can last anywhere from three to five years if they are stored in dark bottles and kept in a cool, dark, dry space. If at any time the liquid begins to separate or smell rancid, discard the bottle.

Syrups: If stored in dark bottles, kept in the refrigerator and with a fresh piece of ginger root added to the liquid, syrups can last up to two months before fermentation sets in and the herbal effectiveness starts to wane.

Ointments/Salves: Herbal ointments/salves can last up to two years before they start to separate or turn rancid as long as they are kept away from moisture and extreme heat. Keep them away from steamy bathrooms and direct heat. You can lengthen the life span of any ointment adding 2-3 drops of benzoin tincture or 10% of jojoba oil to the original mixture and/or storing it in the refrigerator.

Extracted oils: If 20% wheat germ oil is added to the original mixture, the extracted oil can last up to one year before turning rancid or separating. If 3-5 drops of benzoin tincture is added to the original mixture, the oil can last up to 18 months. If 20% jojoba oil is added, extracted oils have been known to last for years.

12. Are dried herbs more potent than fresh herbs or vice versa?

Many herbalists will tell you that fresh herbs are the truest, most potent form to get the most "bang for your buck." However, there are some herbs which actually work best in one form or another. For example, fresh plantain works better than dried plantain as an external poultice for insect bites. However, dried hops is much more potent than fresh hops flowers. Yet, if the "lesser" form of the herb is only available and you need to use it, you can sometimes get moderate results.

13. Is it better to grow your own herbs rather than depend upon store-bought bulk herbs?

Growing herbs from scratch is always better in my opinion because you can regulate the kind of soil and fertilizer. Also important is the fact that by growing your own medicinals, you learn the plant's "personality." While this might sound "woo-woo" to some readers, I assure you that's not my intention. It is one thing to buy an herb at an herb store, seeing only its dried form. It's another thing completely to grow it from seed, and discover what this plant you've been reading or studying about looks like up close and personal. You truly do notice a personality after awhile and, in my opinion, gain a more three dimensional perspective on the herb. However, from a practical point of view, unless you have a large piece of land, the average person cannot grow every single herb they wish to use. Thus, pick five or six you really like and cultivate them in a pot (that is, if they are realistically able to grow in a confined space). For the remainder of your herbs, find a reliable supplier through your local health food/herb store.

14. How safe is it to pick herbs in the wild? Are they better for you?

"Wild crafting," as it is called, is getting harder to do these days since you never know what remote areas have been sprayed with toxic pesticides. I've been out in the boonies where one would never think another human being has trod, and I discover that not only have they trod there, they've also sprayed there! If you are sure no one has sprayed directly over a certain area, find out if any spraying has been done within a quarter mile radius. I say this because if the spraying was done on a windy day, it may have blown over to the "unsprayed area." The other major concern is that you have to be absolutely certain you know what you are picking. Many medicinal herbals are common weeds and many weeds look alike. Because of this, it can be very easy to mistake a healing plant for a look alike plant which is poisonous. Another thing to consider: some medicinal herbs require a specific species be used for best results. I always try to find someone who is familiar with both plants and the area in which they are "wild crafting" before I pick any plant.

15. What if I try an herb and it does not work? Should I use more or discontinue altogether?

There are usually three reasons this could happen. First, you may have picked an herb for the "symptom" instead of the "root" of the problem. A good example of this would be if you had a severe case of food poisoning and you started taking herbs to get rid of the diarrhea. The herbs will probably do nothing for the diarrhea because the root of the problem lies in the intestines where the poison is festering. Attack that area with the appropriate herbal remedy and you automatically also take care of the diarrhea. The second common reason for herbs not doing what "they're supposed to do" is if you attempt to combine them with strong prescription medication. For instance, I have seen cases where people have been addicted to valium and they decide to try an herbal formula which works as a natural sleep aid. If their body is either saturated with valium or they try to take the valium plus the herbal formula, the herbs can actually backfire on them and create the opposite effect: i.e., insomnia. The third reason for herbs not working is very simple: you've picked the wrong herb for your ailment. Again, this goes back to educating yourself on herbal medicine and learning as much as you can about common ailments and the herbs which work best. However, if an herb is not working as it was intended to, do not take more of it to see if "anything happens." My advice would be to see if your situation fits into any of the above three areas and then proceed from there. When you find the right herb for the right problem and you are not interfering with its natural interaction within the body, there's a good chance you will be able to feel some change and get results.

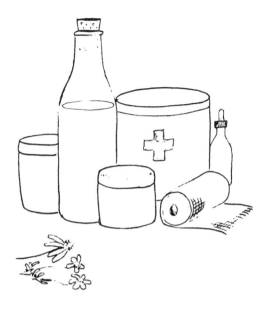

How To Make Your Own Herbal First Aid Kit

Herbal first aid kits are great for the home, office and the car. Below you will find what I consider to be 16 important herbal preparations that one should never be without—especially on long trips.

Regarding the amounts of each preparation for the travel kits, I only take one ounce of the bulk herbs, and 1/2 ounce of the pure essential oils, tinctures and ointments.

The sturdiest carrying cases I have found are plastic tool boxes with the fold-out or removable upper tray. They are durable as well as semi-resistant to heat which is important since herbals need to be kept cool and dry.

Herbal First Aid Kit:

Herb	*Purpose*
Arnica tincture	For external use on sprains.
Homeopathic arnica 30x	For injuries/accidents.
Calendula ointment	Topical treatment for burns and minor skin abrasions.
Calendula tincture	Topical treatment for cold sores and canker sores.
Cayenne powder	Sprinkled on a bleeding cut will help stop blood flow.
Chamomile	Good "calming down" tea.
Comfrey root powder	Mixed with hot water to form a paste, this external poultice can be used for burns or deep cuts to help speed healing.
Echinacea tincture	One teaspoon in 8 oz. of warm water three times a day helps to stop a cold or infection.
Eucalyptus essential oil	Used in a steam inhalation (5-8 drops in a pot of hot water) eucalyptus helps to relieve sinus congestion and respiratory tightness.
Garlic oil capsules	Natural topical disinfectant as well as "portable" internal infection fighting aid for colds and food poisoning. An absolute must when traveling to foreign countries!
Ginger	Excellent tea to improve digestion and soothe an upset stomach. The capsules help to alleviate motion sickness and nausea. Several tablespoons of the dried powder fastened in a drawstring muslin sack and placed in the bathtub helps relieve sore muscles and back pain. Two to three capsules can help stop a headache when they are taken at the onset of the condition.
Lavender essential oil	2-3 drops applied on temples helps to calm anxiety. Great for nervous or rowdy kids. Ten drops in the bath water work to relieve stress and curb insomnia. One to three drops can relieve pain and discomfort from oven burns, minor scrapes and insect bites/stings.
Licorice root	Made into a tea, helps to relieve sore throats, loosen phlegm and raise blood sugar levels.

Peppermint essential oil	2-3 drops applied on temples relieves headaches and wakes one up during long trips. Ten drops in the bath water help to "perk one up" when tired.
Peppermint leaves	Taken in a tea, soothes indigestion.
Red Raspberry leaves	Taken hot, the tea helps one at the onset of colds and flu. Taken cold, the tea works to stop diarrhea.
White Willow Bark	Natural headache/body ache tea.

This may seem to be a lot of stuff. However, if you only carry one ounce portions of each dried herb and half ounce bottles of the essential oils, tinctures and ointments, your herbal first aid kit can be quite compact. One word of advice: Do not use plastic storage bottles or plastic bags. When heat hits the plastic, the plastic can soften which can affect the herbs. Plastic bags can also trap moisture or change the flavor of the herbal tea. Never use plastic bottles to store pure essential oils since the concentrated oil will melt the plastic! Small glass bottles are best, however, people are often concerned about breaking them. You can't avoid glass bottles with the pure essential oils, but for the dried herbs, try using small brown paper bags, securing the contents with a rubber band. Finally, to make sure your first aid kit stays fresh and medicinally potent, add a new batch of bulk herbs every six months. The pure essential oils, tinctures and ointments should be replaced every one to three years.

QUICK & EASY REFERENCE CHART FOR COMMON AILMENTS

The following 12 pages contain a reference chart for common ailments. Check individual chapters for any cautions that may apply to you.

AILMENT	HERB(S)	FORM	ACTION	PAGE
Acne	calendula	tea	blood & liver cleanser	19
	chamomile (external application only)	steam inhalation (dried herb)	loosens toxins from pores	38
	dandelion	tea	excellent liver cleanser	50
	juniper (external application only)	steam inhalation (5-8 drops of essential oil)	loosens toxins from pores	99
	lavender (external application only)	essential oil (one drop on pimple)	helps to dry up pimple	105
Anxiety	chamomile	tea	calms the mind and nerves	35
	juniper	bath (10-15 drops of essential oil)	centers mind & body	99
Backache	cascara sagrada	tea (when related to constipation)	relieves pressure if colon is impacted	22
	cayenne (external application only)	extracted oil, liniment	warms the area, stimulates circulation	33
	chamomile (external application only)	essential oil (3-4 drops rubbed into back muscles)	relaxes tense muscles and soothes pain	39
	dong quai	tea or extract (when related to female problems)	warms body and relieves spasms	54
	elder (internal & external application)	tincture (10-20 drops in water or used straight as a liniment)	allows better movement, lessens pain	66
	ginger (external application only)	bath (dried herb)	generates heat, stimulates circulation, lessens pain	81
	lavender (external application only)	essential oil (4 drops to 1 tablespoon of base oil)	calms & soothes muscles	106

AILMENT	HERB(S)	ACTION	FORM	PAGE
Bed Wetting	St. John's Wort	calms, helps relieve nervous tension	extract or tincture	138
Body Aches	cayenne (external application only)	warms the area, stimulates circulation	extracted oil, liniment	33
	eucalyptus (external application only)	cools, penetrates muscles to relieve pain	bath (10-15 drops of essential oil)	71
	ginger (external application only)	generates heat, stimulates circulation, lessens pain	bath (dried herb)	81
Bleeding	calendula (external application only)	contracts blood vessels	tincture	18
Blood Poisoning	cayenne (internal & external application)	coagulates blood	dried herb	30
	echinacea	cleanses lymph glands, purifies blood	tea or tincture	61
	plantain (internal & external application)	pulls poison and pain from area	tea or fresh leaf/ dried herb poultice	127
Bruises	arnica	taken immediately; can reduce swelling and pain	homeopathic tablets (6x or 30x potency)	12
	St. John's Wort (external application only)	reduces inflammation beneath the skin	extracted oil	133
Burns	calendula (external application only)	takes "heat" out of burn, speeds healing	ointment	16
	chamomile (external application only)	soothes, cools and speeds healing	essential oil (3-4 drops on burn)	39
	comfrey (external application only)	"feeds" cells and regenerates them, heals tissue	ointment or poultice	44
	elder (external application only)	eases pain	ointment (in coconut oil base)	67

173

AILMENT	HERB(S)	FORM	ACTION	PAGE
Burns	lavender (external application only)	essential oil (2-3 drops on burn)	takes "heat" out of burn, speeds healing	104
	St. John's Wort (external application only)	extracted oil	reduces inflammation & pain, speeds healing	133
	white willow (external application only)	poultice	soothing, "cools" burn	144
Circulation (Sluggish)	cayenne (internal & external application)	tea, bath (dried herb)	generates tremendous heat throughout body	32
	ginger (internal & external application)	tea, bath (dried herb)	generates heat, activates body's circulation	82
	lavender (external application only)	essential oil (5-8 drops in foot bath)	encourages and activates circulation	106
Colds & Flu	catnip	tea	unlocks toxins and soothes nerves	26
	cayenne	tea, bath (dried herb)	stimulates circulation, unlocks toxins	32
	echinacea	tea, tincture	blood & lymph cleanser/natural antibiotic	59
	elder	tea (with equal parts of peppermint)	promotes perspiration to unlock toxins	64
	eucalyptus	bath (10-15 drops of essential oil)	soothes aching muscles, clears sinuses	69
	garlic	fresh cloves, oil capsules	anti-bacterial, anti-viral, anti-fungal, anti-parasitic	74
	ginger	tea, bath (dried herb)	pulls toxins from the pores, soothes aches	82

174

AILMENT	HERB(S)	FORM	ACTION	PAGE
Colds & Flu	red raspberry	tea	tonic for the body, cleanses liver, vitamin-rich	130
Colic	catnip	diluted tea for babies, enema	dispels gas	25
	chamomile	tea, fomentation	dispels gas	36
Constipation	cascara sagrada (strong action)	tea	tones bowels, encourages peristalsis action	20
	chamomile (mild action)	tea	softens stool	36
	dong quai (very mild action)	tea or extract	relieves tension and spasms in the colon	53
Cough	juniper (external application only)	steam inhalation (5-8 drops of essential oil)	soothes cough	99
	lavender (external application only)	steam inhalation (5-8 drops of essential oil)	helps kill infection, relieve congestion	105
	licorice	tea	loosens phlegm, soothes throat	107
	plantain	tea, syrup	breaks up congestion & loosens phlegm	124
Diarrhea	catnip	tea	natural antibiotic, soothes entire body	26
	ginger	tea	dispels gas, aids in digestion	83
	red raspberry	tea (taken cold)	astringent	130

175

AILMENT	HERB(S)	FORM	ACTION	PAGE
Dizziness	lavender (external application only)	essential oil (3-5 drops sniffed on cotton ball)	calming, soothes hysteria	105
	peppermint (external application only)	strong tea, essential oil (3-5 drops sniffed on cotton ball)	perks up the senses, clears the mind	119
Earache	elder	tea (taken with equal parts of peppermint when cold symptoms are present)	through eliminating toxins, relieves pressure	65
	garlic	extracted oil (placed directly into ear)	kills infection, natural antibiotic	77
Female Complaints:				
Menstruation	catnip	tea	relieves cramps, promotes menstruation	26
	chamomile	tea	hot tea relieves cramping, cold tea promotes menstruation	37
	dong quai	tea, extract	regulates cycle, promotes menstruation, reduces bloating, soothes body aches	53
	juniper (external application only)	essential oil (3-4 drops to 1 tablespoon of base oil)	relieves cramps when oil is rubbed on abdomen, promotes menstruation	100
	lavender (external application only)	essential oil (4 drops to 1 tablespoon of base oil)	relieves cramps when oil is rubbed on abdomen	106

AILMENT	HERB(S)	ACTION	FORM	PAGE
Female Complaints:				
Menstruation	parsley	promotes menstruation	tea	113
	peppermint	stops or decreases flow	tea	119
	red raspberry	decreases flow	tea	130
Menopause	dong quai	hormone balancer, can be used to wean oneself off estrogen replacement therapy	tea, extract	55
PMS	dong quai	decreases bloating, breast soreness and emotional distress	tea, extract	55
	juniper (external application only)	calms & soothes jangled nerves	bath (10-15 drops of essential oil)	99
	lavender (external application only)	relieves tension, aids in restful sleep	bath (10-15 drops of essential oil)	103
Fever	catnip	calms as it brings down fever	tea, enema	26
	elder	best when fever is hot & dry, promotes perspiration	tea (with equal parts of peppermint)	64
	eucalyptus (external application only)	"cools" the body while clearing congestion	bath (15-20 drops of essential oil)	71
	lavender (external application only)	reduces "hot" conditions as it calms nerves	bath (10-15 drops of essential oil) 2-3 drops of essential oil on wet washcloth	106
	white willow	anti-inflammatory, reduces aches & pains	tea	142

177

AILMENT	HERB(S)	FORM	ACTION	PAGE
Headache	cascara sagrada	tea (when related to constipation)	loosens & eliminates toxic debris in bowel	22
	ginger (internal & external application)	2-3 caps at onset of headache (internal), foot bath (external)	best for stress headaches, stimulates circulation	81
	lavender (external application only)	essential oil (3 drops rubbed on back of neck)	calms & soothes, promotes sleep	105
	peppermint (internal & external application)	tea, essential oil (2-3 drops rubbed on temples), 2-3 drops of essential oil on wet washcloth	"cools" the head, clears the sinuses, reduces pain	117
	white willow	tea	anti-inflammatory, soothes entire body	142
Indigestion	catnip	tea	breaks up gas	26
	chamomile	tea	soothes gas pains (esp. when centered around navel)	36
	ginger	tea	settles the stomach & encourages digestion	83
	parsley	tea	helps body assimilate food and minerals	114
	peppermint	tea	stimulates liver/promotes digestive juices	119
Infection	echinacea	tea, tincture	cleanses blood & lymph glands	60

AILMENT	HERB(S)	FORM	ACTION	PAGE
Infection	garlic (internal & external application)	fresh cloves, oil capsules	"natural antibiotic" cleanses blood as it kills germs	75
Inflammation	arnica (internal & external application)	homeopathic tablets (internal only—6x or 30 x potency), tincture (external)	reduces swelling if administered immediately	12
	chamomile (internal & external application)	tea, essential oil (3-4 drops straight or mixed with 1 tablespoon of base oil)	soothes nerves as it reduces puffiness	39
	elder	poultice (dried flowers mixed with equal parts chamomile flowers)	soothes and cools area, reduces soreness	67
	licorice	tea	coats sore throat, encourages mucus release	108
	St. John's Wort (external application only)	tincture or extracted oil	reduces nerve pain and damage	134
	white willow	tea	soothes & reduces swollen joints	142
Insect Bites	eucalyptus (external application only)	essential oil (one teaspoon to one cup warm water)	repels insects	71
	juniper	tea, berry poultice (to draw out infection)	clears poisons out of bloodstream via urinary tract as a topical, pulls poison out of bite	98
	lavender (external application only)	essential oil (1-2 drops undiluted on bite/sting)	reduces pain & swelling	105

179

AILMENT	HERB(S)	FORM	ACTION	PAGE
Insect Bites	parsley (external application only)	poultice (fresh or dried leaves), juice (repels insects)	poultice reduces pain & swelling	115
	plantain (external application only)	poultice (fresh leaves applied to bite/sting)	pulls out poison, reduces swelling in minutes	124
Insomnia	catnip	tea	soothes the nerves (great for kids)	25
	chamomile	tea	soothes jangled nerves, irritability & anger	35
	dong quai (mild effect)	tea, extract	"warms" the body, creating calm	53
	hops	tea, bath (dried herbs)	gently sedates without narcotic side effects	93
	lavender	tea, bath (using dried herb or 10-15 drops of essential oil), essential oil (2-3 drops on pillowcase)	aromatic scent is legendary for promoting sleep	103
Nausea & Vomiting	ginger	tea	calms & settles stomach	81
Nerves	chamomile	tea	soothes nervous stomach and calms entire system	37
	hops	tea	gently sedates without narcotic side effects	93

180

HEAD(S)	FORM	ACTION	PAGE
Nerves juniper (external application only)	bath (10-15 drops of essential oil)	reduces nervous tension (esp. good for those who absorb negative emotions from others)	99
lavender (external application only)	tea, bath (using dried herb or 10-15 drops of essential oil)	soothes externally, aromatic scent promotes calm	104
Pain (general) ginger (internally)	capsule (500-3000 milligrams/day)	helps relieve acute & even chronic pain	83
Rash dandelion (if related to toxic liver)	tea	cleanses the liver, discharging trapped poisons	50
peppermint (if poison ivy/oak)	bath (10-15 drops of essential oil)	cools the rash	121
plantain	tea, fresh leaf poultice, skin wash	pulls out poison from bloodstream, cools the rash	127
Sinus chamomile (external application only)	steam inhalation (dried herb)	aromatic fumes are mildly anti-bacterial	38
eucalyptus (external application only)	steam inhalation (5-8 drops of essential oil)	inhaled, the vapors are strongly anti-viral	70
garlic	fresh cloves, oil capsule	natural antibiotic properties kill infection	74
parsley	tea	clears built-up toxins and releases congestion	114
peppermint (external application only)	steam inhalation (5-8 drops of essential oil)	opens up sinuses, clears head	120

181

AILMENT	HERB(S)	ACTION	FORM	PAGE
Skin Ulcers	comfrey (external application only)	"knits" skin together & promotes cell regeneration	poultice	45
	hops (external application only)	soothing with mild antibiotic abilities	poultice	94
	plantain (internal & external application)	cools & soothes as it pulls out infection and heals	tea, poultice (fresh leaf works best)	126
	white willow (external application only)	high tannin content in bark is a mild astringent	skin wash	144
Sore Throat	cayenne	natural antiseptic, pain relief and loosens mucus	gargle	32
	echinacea (strep throat)	antibiotic action may stop infection from spreading	tea, tincture	60
	eucalyptus (external application only)	aromatic vapors have anti-viral properties	steam inhalation (5-8 drops of essential oil)	70
	licorice	coats & soothes throat as it loosens mucus	tea	108
Sprains	arnica	when used immediately, can eliminate swelling	homeopathic tablets (6x or 30x potency), tincture (external application only)	14
	cayenne (external application only)	stimulates circulation to affected area	extracted oil, liniment	33
	chamomile (external application only)	soothes & "cools" the pain, reduces swelling	extracted oil	38

182

	Herb	Form	Action	Page
Sprains	comfrey	*homeopathic tablets or tincture in 30x potency, poultice (dried root or fresh leaves)	helps speed healing to tissue, muscle & tendons	42
Stomach Ache	chamomile	tea	soothes while reducing any gastric inflammation	37
Teething Pain	chamomile	**homeopathic tablets (3x potency)	reduces pain while calming restlessness and whining	40
Wounds	calendula (external application only)	ointment	anti-inflammatory, soothes & "cools"	16
	catnip (for minor wounds)	poultice (fresh plant is best)	acts as a natural antibiotic	27
	comfrey (external application only)	ointment, poultice	speeds healing with its cell regeneration ability	45
	echinacea (external application only)	extract, ointment	prevents infection—especially when pus is present	61
	garlic (topical antibiotic)	fresh cloves, oil capsule	natural antibiotic and disinfectant	77
	lavender (external application only)	essential oil (1-2 drops)	kills harmful bacteria & speeds healing	104
	peppermint (external application only)	essential oil (2 drops)	extremely antiseptic, "cooling"	120
	plantain (external application only)	fresh leaf poultice	coagulates blood/promotes fast healing	125
	St. John's Wort (external application only)	extracted oil, tincture	reduces pain & inflammation, fights infection	134
	white willow (external application only)	poultice (bleeding wounds)	astringent, "cooling"	143

*Homeopathic comfrey is found under the name Symphytum

**Homeopathic chamomile is found under the name Chamomilla

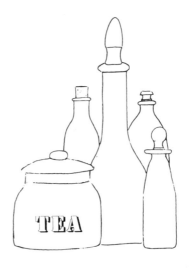

HOW TO MAKE HERBAL STUFF

Here are detailed descriptions on how to make the various preparations described in the herbal chapters.

INFUSION

The most common way to make an herbal tea. The medicinal properties are extracted in water by a more gentle process. An infusion is generally used for the more delicate parts of a plant (i.e., the flowers and leaves). Hot (NOT boiling) water is poured over the herb. The mixture is then allowed to steep for 10-20 minutes.

A cold infusion may also be called for. This requires pouring cold water over the herbs and allowing the mixture to stand, covered, overnight.

The suggested tea to water ratio for an infusion is: one heaping teaspoon of the dried herb or two heaping teaspoons of the fresh herb to 8 oz. of distilled water.

DECOCTION

A decoction is required when using the "tougher" plant parts (i.e., roots, barks, berries, leaf buds, nuts). Boiling water is necessary to extract the medicinal essence from the core. The herb is

usually placed into cold water and brought to a boil. The mixture is
then allowed to simmer for 10-20 minutes (or longer if indicated).
The harder the plant material, the longer it will take for the medicinal
elements to be released.

The suggested tea to water ratio for a decoction is two heaping
tablespoons of the dried herb to 12 oz. of cold distilled water. Note:
Once the herb has simmered for 10-20 minutes, you will end up
with less water than you started with due to the evaporation process.

EXTRACT

An extract is similar to a decoction in that the herb is boiled.
However, the extract requires one to boil the plant on low heat for a
long period of time, allowing the liquid to almost evaporate before
adding additional liquid. Extracts can be made with distilled water,
alcohol or glycerin, depending upon which solvent interacts best
with the chosen herb. They are very concentrated. While one can
make herbal extracts at home, they can be tricky for the beginning
herbal student to gauge. For this reason, I tend to lean more toward
trusted commercial extracts. The suggested dose for an extract is
one-half to one teaspoon of the extract given straight or in distilled
water.

TINCTURE

A tincture can be one of the most convenient ways to take
herbs—aside from capsules and tablets. Herbal tinctures are made
with either 80 proof or 190 proof alcohol (known as "grain
alcohol"). There are also natural vegetable glycerine tinctures.
Glycerine tinctures are considered best for internal use—especially
for children under the age of 12. Yet, with vegetable glycerine-based
tinctures, one needs to *double* the necessary dose. Alcohol-based
tinctures should be used regardless when the herb in question is
resinous or oily in nature. Herbs of this kind need alcohol to extract
their active principles. If a tincture is alcohol-based and you don't
want to ingest a lot of alcohol into your body, you can put the
tincture dose into 8 oz. of boiling water, thus, evaporating much of
the alcohol content.

Tinctures are very potent. One ounce of a tincture equals the
potency of one ounce of the powdered herb. Thus, six to eight
drops placed under the tongue or put into 8 oz. of hot water is
equivalent to one cup of tea.

To be quite honest, I have never been able to make an effective homemade glycerine tincture. When I need a glycerine tincture, I buy it at my local herb store. Thus, the following recipe is for an *alcohol* tincture. Substituting vegetable glycerine in place of the alcohol *will not* work.

The suggested herb to alcohol ratio is as follows: Four ounces **dried** herbs **OR** eight ounces of **fresh** herbs to 16 ounces of 80 proof vodka or grain alcohol. Combine the herbs and alcohol into a wide mouthed, glass bottle. I have found that pickle jars and mayonnaise jars work well for this purpose. Always allow enough room in the bottle so that the herbs and alcohol are not packed right to the top. Twist the lid tightly and shake vigorously. Place the bottle in a cool, dark place for 14 days. Three times each day, shake the bottle so that the contents have a chance to move around. On the 14th day, strain the liquid through a clean muslin cloth. Once all the liquid has been emptied, twist the muslin cloth tightly to force out the remaining tincture. Store the tincture in a dark bottle and keep it in a dark, cool cupboard. The mixture should last 2-3 years, depending upon how it is stored and what particular solvent was used in the extraction process (i.e., alcohol-based tinctures last longer than glycerin-based tinctures).

SYRUP

Homemade herbal cough syrups are as old as time. To make the syrup, first make either an infusion or decoction, depending upon if the herb you are using falls into the flower/leaf category or the root/bark/berry/nuts category. Use two cups of distilled water and follow the same herb to water measurements (i.e., an infusion calls for one heaping teaspoon of the dried herb or two heaping teaspoons of the fresh herb to 8 oz. of distilled water. For the syrup, simply double the measurements to meet the two cup criteria). Allow the infusion or decoction to cook down to half its original volume (i.e., one cup of liquid should remain). This usually takes about 30-45 minutes. Take liquid off the heat, strain out the herbs and gradually stir in two cups of raw honey (I find tupelo honey works great). Bring the mixture to a slight boil and take off the heat again. Add one or two "thumb-size" chunks of fresh ginger root to the syrup. This helps preserve the syrup and catalyze the herb. Let the mixture slightly cool before placing it into a dark, corked bottle for storage. NOTE: the bottle must be corked since screw-capped bottles may explode if any fermentation takes place. Store the syrup in the refrigerator. It should keep for 4-6 weeks.

THE FOLLOWING HERBAL PREPARATIONS ARE FOR EXTERNAL USE ONLY.

LINIMENT

Herbal liniments are great when you need to add a burst of external circulation to sore muscles and aching joints. An herbal liniment can be made two ways. The first way is to combine 1 1/2 cups of the dried herb to two cups of inexpensive vodka or pure apple cider vinegar. Put the herbs and vodka/cider vinegar in a large dark glass bottle and shake vigorously. Keep the mixture in a cool, dark cupboard for 7-11 days, shaking the mixture at least twice a day. After 7-11 days, strain the herbs and add 1-2 tablespoons of olive oil. The olive oil helps to more easily spread the liniment over the area being treated. Before using, always shake the bottle to distribute the olive oil.

The second way to make a liniment involves the use of pure essential oils. This version requires no "incubation" period as mentioned above. Simply fill a bottle with 8 oz. of vodka and add 40-50 drops of whatever essential oil you wish you use. Don't substitute apple cider vinegar this time because the vinegar will not blend well with the aromatic essential oils. It is best to use the essential oil blend within one week of making it since the essential oils loose their aromatic "punch."

For both types of liniments, use gentle but persistent friction against the skin. The liniment should be rubbed into the skin with a brisk motion so that all of it is absorbed.

FOMENTATION

Not to be confused with *fermentation*. A fomentation is a fancy term for saying "a cloth soaked in liquid." One would use a fomentation on somebody who has pain or inflammation. To make a fomentation, you will need a clean, cotton cloth (flannel is best). An herbal tea is brewed up to three times the normal strength. The cloth is then soaked in the tea liquid, wrung out and—once the burning heat disperses—is placed across or around the affected area to be treated. Retaining the heat is important with fomentations since it is the moist heat which aids in the treatment. For this reason, placing plastic wrap over the hot, herb-soaked cotton cloth is recommended. Once the cloth becomes cool, remove, re-soak in the hot tea liquid and repeat. Note: If the area to be treated is swollen due to a sprain or break, use cold, NOT HOT fomentations and see a doctor immediately!

POULTICE

This is one of the most effective forms of external herbal relief. A poultice can be made many different ways, but here are two of the more common approaches.

When using fresh herbs, you can either lightly heat the indicated plant's flowers or leaves in a sieve until moist or simply bruise (rub the leaves or flowers between your palms) or macerate (lightly chew until moist but not into a ball) and apply the plant directly to the area that needs to be treated. Hold the fresh herbal poultice on the area with your palm or cover it with a cloth or masking tape to keep it in place. Hold in place as needed.

The second way to make a poultice is using dried herbs. To make life easier, you'll want to grind the dried herbs into a granulated or fine powder form. The amount of herbs needed will depend upon the size of the area you want to treat. For an average size poultice (3"x3") combine 2-4 tablespoons of the dried, powdered herb with enough hot water to make a thick paste. To give the poultice more consistency, add a teaspoon of honey and a teaspoon of olive oil. (Wheat germ oil, safflower oil or peanut oil can be substituted). Stir the contents briskly until the mixture is smooth and uniform. (You might want to flip it between your palms, as you would a meat patty, in order to knead the contents together). Immediately apply this mixture to the affected area and cover with plastic wrap to hold it in place. If heat is required, a moist heat pad is preferred. However, a regular heat pad or hot water bottle will do. Usually, a dried herb poultice is left on 4-8 hours. When it is removed, it must NOT be reused.

Generally, poultices are used to draw out infections, inflammations and poisons (such as insect bites).

OINTMENT/SALVE

This is one of the oldest ways herbs were used externally in days gone by. Usually, ointments/salves are used for their emollient, protective and healing effects. It can be a messy job to make an ointment/salve at home but, often times, the specific herbal ointment/salve you need is either unavailable on the commercial market or difficult to find. Thus, making it yourself is the only way. Here's how:

Use a Pyrex or stainless steel saucepan. Buy inexpensive wooden spoons for stirring. Plastic will not work because they melt with the heat. You will need a one quart glass jelly jar for straining the ointment into and smaller glass containers for storing the ointment. Once again, plastic jars will not work since the hot oil will melt the sides. Finally, a muslin cloth cut approximately 16"x16" will be necessary to fit over the one quart glass jelly jar for use in straining and separating the herb particles from the oil. (A muslin drawstring "jelly bag" using for canning is actually your best bet, but they are often hard to find).

To make approximately 12-14 oz. of an ointment/salve, you will need 16 oz. of lard or olive oil, 2 oz. of beeswax, 2 oz. of the dried herbs OR 4 oz. of the finely cut fresh herb and one-half teaspoon of benzoin tincture as a preservative. I know that lard sounds awful and please feel free to replace it with either straight olive oil or equal parts olive oil and safflower oil. Do not use canola oil for any medicinal herbal preparations since it can clog pores and even cause blackheads. Over the years, herbalists have discovered that lard extracts more of the herb's medicinal benefit and effectively draws the healing potential into the skin when the ointment/salve is applied. However, lard often smells bad, sometimes doesn't absorb completely into the skin and often does not keep as long as the olive oil variety. My personal preference when I make salves is always olive oil. However, go ahead and experiment with both options and see which one you like the best.

If you are using lard, melt it on very low heat stove-top. Once liquid, add the herbs. If you are using olive oil and/or safflower oil, combine the herb(s) and oil in a saucepan and heat the mixture stove-top on low. Keep covered so the herbal oils do not escape into the air. However, stir and "pumice" the mixture with a wooden spoon every ten minutes or so to make sure the herbs are saturated with the lard or olive oil. Continue for two hours, making sure the mixture never gets so hot that it starts to burn.

The idea is to gently pull the medicinal qualities out of the plants. If you cook the mixture too fast, the healing volatile oils are extracted too quickly and are often "burned out" of the mixture. Your final ointment/salve product will smell like burnt grass and quite frankly, I don't feel it has the best medicinal benefit. You have to be cautious of overcooking any herb, but you have to really watch it with flowers and leaves (such as chamomile and plantain) since they are delicate to begin with. What I like to do with more delicate plant material is bring the mixture just to a boil and then turn off the heat, letting the oil sit covered for 20 minutes. Then, turn the burner on low again and repeat the process. You don't have to stare at the stuff the whole time, but please don't leave it unattended since these mixtures have been known to pop, explode and even voluntarily catch on fire when they get too hot and are not stirred.

After two hours of cooking, the plants should look darker. Turn off the heat and cover the pot. If you are using olive oil as your base, allow the mixture to sit covered for up to eight hours. If you are using lard, you'll have to strain the herbs right away since lard congeals when cooled. Before straining either mixture, gently melt two oz. of beeswax in the one quart glass jelly jar. You can use a double boiler to melt the beeswax or place the jar in the oven, using no more than 180° F. of heat.

Once the beeswax has melted, secure the 16"x16" muslin cloth around the neck of the jar with a rubber band and slowly strain the herbal oil through the cloth. (If your base is olive oil, you will have to heat the mixture first so it will melt evenly into the beeswax). To make sure all the oil has been extracted from the herbs, carefully remove the muslin cloth and squeeze it tightly until the last drop is forced through the herbs. Stir the mixture to make sure the beeswax is blended and then, as a preservative, add one teaspoon of benzoin tincture. You can now pour the liquid ointment into separate glass jars for storage. However, you will need to do it quickly because the ointment and beeswax will start to harden within minutes. When the ointment cools, tightly secure the jars and store them in a dark cupboard or in the refrigerator. The ointment/salve will usually last up to one year before separating and turning rancid. Once that happens, it is best to throw it out and do the whole thing over again.

HERBAL OIL EXTRACTION

This is not to be confused with the pure essential herbal oils which are steam distilled. This herbal oil is used more as an external rub (much like a liniment). The healing essence of the herb is extracted from the herb using heat. An herbal oil extraction can be made two ways.

The first way is done when you need the oil right away and can't wait around for it to "mature." Combine one part dried herb by weight to eight parts by volume of olive oil, grapeseed oil, safflower oil or a combination of any of those three. In other words, one ounce (by weight) of the dried herb to eight ounces (by volume) of the oil. If you are using fresh herbs, the herb to oil ratio is one part fresh herbs by weight to four ounces by volume of the oil. Adding three tablespoons of wheat germ oil to the blend will act as a natural "preservative" and make the oil last longer. Stir the oil and herb together in a stainless steel or Pyrex saucepan. Heat the mixture at a very low temperature, stirring constantly. You DO NOT want to heat the oil too fast because you can burn the herbs as well as start a grease fire! Allow the oil and herbs to gently simmer for 10 minutes, then turn off the burner. Cover and let it be for about 30 minutes. Re-heat the liquid, stirring constantly, until it starts to simmer again. Let it simmer for 5-10 minutes on low heat, turn off the burner and cover. You can repeat this two or three times more, depending upon how strong you want the oil extraction. Obviously, the more you let the hot oil blend with the herbs, the better. I've kept this going for up to 12 hours with great results. However, the more the liquid is simmered, the more it will evaporate. When you're finished, strain out the herbal sediment through a muslin cloth and pour the hot herbal oil into a dark, amber glass jar. Although it is optional, stirring in one-half teaspoon of benzoin tincture will make the oil last longer before turning rancid. Allow the mixture to cool at room temperature. Store the herbal oil extract in a dark, cool cupboard. It should last 6-18 months.

You'll need both patience and time to make an herbal oil extract the old fashioned way. But if you don't need it right away, I think the following process produces a much better oil with fuller herbal powers. The ratio of herbs to oil (weight to volume) is the same as mentioned above. Include the three tablespoons of wheat germ oil in addition for "preservative" powers. Pack a wide mouthed glass canning jar three-quarters of the way full with the fresh or dried herbs and pour the required amount of oil over them. Make sure the canning jar has a wide enough opening so the herbs can come out easily once the oil is ready to "harvest." Tightly close the lid. Shake the bottle so that the contents are thoroughly mixed together, then place the canning jar directly in the sun or on a windowsill so that the sun shines directly on it for at least three hours each day. Every day, shake this mixture at least twice to circulate the herbs and oil. You can unscrew the lid occasionally to test the oil's texture and smell, but try to keep it to a minimum since the least amount of air getting into the bottle, the better it will be.

One important note here: when using fresh herbs, before placing them into the canning jar, put them into a bowl and sprinkle enough 80 proof vodka or grain alcohol over the plant to lightly saturate it. Set it aside for 3-6 hours and then pack the herb into the jar and pour the oil over it. In addition, place several layers of a muslin cloth over the canning jar and secure tightly. The reason for the muslin is that if you place an airtight lid over fresh herbs and oil, the natural water from within the plant can breed bacteria. The alcohol pre-soak helps alleviate part of this problem, but the muslin allows for evaporation. Before I figured this out, I ruined lots of good fresh herbal oils due to spoilage. You can tell if a fresh herbal oil is spoiled when you open the lid and need to step back about 40 feet because the smell is so wicked. If your fresh herbal oil spoils, you have no choice but to throw it away and start over.

Now, back to the shaking of the jar. Some people only keep this routine up for 2-3 weeks before harvesting the oil. That's okay, but if you can wait a full six or even twelve weeks, you will have a much richer herbal blend. When you harvest the oil, either strain the herbs through a plastic strainer or through a clean, muslin cloth. The muslin cloth is better since you can hand press every last drop of the oil. (Remember, the strainer should be plastic or stainless steel— NOT aluminum). Adding a half teaspoon of benzoin tincture helps the oil last longer. Place the strained oil into an amber glass jar and store it in a dark, cool spot. This oil can last up to 18 months.

STEAM INHALATION

An herbal inhalation is a great way to clear congestion from the bronchial tubes and lungs and can help soothe sore throats. Fresh herbs, dried herbs or pure essential oils are used. However, I feel essential oils are the most effective way to benefit from this herbal treatment.

Fill a large pot (pasta pots work well) with tap water and bring it to a rolling boil. Set the pot aside. Situate yourself in a comfortable position in front of the covered pot and drape a towel over your head to form a "tent". Now, place your herbs into the water OR 5-8 drops of the pure essential oil. Inhale the herbal fumes deeply, taking care not to get so close to the steam that you burn your skin or interior nasal passage. Continue for 10-20 minutes. If you are using essential oils, they will evaporate within five minutes. When this happens, simply add 5-8 more drops into the hot water.

HERBAL SPRAY

Natural herbal sprays are easy and inexpensive to make. Fill an 8 ounce plastic or glass spray bottle with 7 ounce of cold distilled water. To this mixture, add 50-100 drops of any pure essential oil. Shake vigorously before using and spray freely around sick rooms to disinfect as well as create a pleasant aromatic environment. The herbal spray usually lasts up to one month before losing its aromatic and healing power.

BIBLIOGRAPHY & REFERENCE

In addition to listing my reference sources, I have also included a brief description of the material.

Brown, Tom. *Tom Brown's Guide to Wild Edible and Medicinal Plants.* New York: Berkley Books, 1985.

(Brown gives both medicinal advice on 44 plants as well as his own outdoor experiences with the plants. His unique approach with plants is physical, mental and spiritual).

Castleman, Michael. *The Healing Herbs.* Pennsylvania: Rodale Press, 1991.

(Castleman covers 100 herbs, including their history and current use. Very conservative "facts only" approach. Good reference guide for anyone interested in herbs).

Christopher, John R., N.D., M.H. Natural Healing Newsletter: "American Indian Herbs" (Volume 4, No. 11). Springville, Utah: Christopher Publications, 1983.

————. Natural Healing Newsletter: "Arthritis, A Needless Crippler" (Volume 3, No. 11). Springville, Utah: Christopher Publications, 1982.

————. Natural Healing Newsletter: "Bone, Flesh and Cartilage" (Volume 1, No. 8). Springville, Utah: Christopher Publications, 1980.

————. Natural Healing Newsletter: "Curative Comfrey" (Volume 4, No. 3). Springville, Utah: Christopher Publications, 1983.

————. Natural Healing Newsletter: "Garlic: Man's Best Friend In A Toxic World" (Volume 2, No. 9). Springville, Utah: Christopher Publications, 1981.

————. Natural Healing Newsletter: "Herbal First Aid—Part I" (Volume 3, No. 1). Springville, Utah: Christopher Publications, 1982.

————. Natural Healing Newsletter: "Herbal First Aid—Part II" (Volume 3, No. 1). Springville, Utah: Christopher Publications, 1982.

————. Natural Healing Newsletter: "Licorice: The Legendary Herb" (Volume 3, No. 3). Springville, Utah: Christopher Publications, 1982.

————. Natural Healing Newsletter: "Oak Bark" (Volume 2, No. 10). Springville, Utah: Christopher Publications, 1981.

————. Natural Healing Newsletter: "Pain Palliatives" (Volume 4, No. 5). Springville, Utah: Christopher Publications, 1983.

————. Natural Healing Newsletter: "Ten Honorable Herbs" (Volume 4, No. 7). Springville, Utah: Christopher Publications, 1983.

————. Natural Healing Newsletter: "The Ten Most Important Herbs" (Volume 1, No. 3). Springville, Utah: Christopher Publications, 1980.

(Ten newsletters in a series of over 70 which offer further detailed information on herbs and their specific uses. Good easy-to-read reference material).

————. Dr. Christopher's New Herb Lectures—Audio tape series. Springville, Utah: Christopher Publications, 1978.

(Over ten hours of Dr. Christopher speaking on everything from the basics of herbal medicine to herbal formulas. Good for anyone who wants to really understand the field of herbology).

————. School of Natural Healing. Springville, Utah: Christopher Publications, 1992 (Tenth Printing).

(Considered THE reference volume for herbalists. Best suited for those who have a basic understanding of herbs).

Esplan, Ceres. Herbal Teas For Health and Healing. Rochester, Vermont: Healing Arts Press, 1988.

(Brief overview of medicinal herbs. Minor reference guide for anyone new to medicinal herbs).

Evelyn, Nancy. The Herbal Medicine Chest. Freedom, California: The Crossing Press, 1986.

(A good reference guide for the student which covers about two dozen herbs and oils and their various uses).

Heinerman, John. Heinerman's Encyclopedia of Fruits, Vegetables and Herbs. New York: Parker Publishing Company, 1988.

(A good reference guide for both beginner and practitioner which covers not only herbs but medicinal fruits and vegetables).

Hutchens, Alma R. *The Handbook of Native American Herbs.* Massachusetts: Shambhala Publications, 1992.

(Brief medicinal overview of over 100 herbs used by Native Americans. Includes some formulas and folklore).

Jackson, Mildred, N.D. & Teague, Terri, N.D., D.C. *The Handbook of Alternatives to Chemical Medicine.* Oakland, California: Lawton-Teague Publications, 1991 (16th printing).

(An "everything but the kitchen sink" guide to herbs, with hundreds of formulas and preparations. Also includes basic emergency medical procedures and a useful vitamin chart).

Jensen, Bernard, Ph.D. *Herbs: Wonder Healers.* Escondido, California: Bernard Jensen, Publisher, 1992.

(Includes everything from herbs to edible grasses. Emphasis is on re-building the body through nutrition and plants. The text jumps around a bit but it is still a good reference guide for both the student and the practitioner).

Kloss, Jethro. *Back to Eden.* Loma Linda, California: Back to Eden Books Publishing Company, 1992 (11th printing).

(Considered by many herbalists to be "THE herb bible." One of the most definitive books written on herbs. Includes tons of information on nutrition and general health).

Lee, William H., D.Sc., R.Ph. & Lee, Lynn, CN. *The Book of Practical Aromatherapy.* Connecticut: Keats Publishing, 1992.

(A good reference guide for the student and practitioner of aromatherapy. Includes interesting history and application on dozens of pure essential oils).

Lucas, Richard M. *Miracle Medicine Herbs.* New York: Parker Publishing Company, 1991.

(Well-researched herbal guide with plenty of scientific data and testimonials to back up medicinal claims).

Lust, John. *The Herb Book.* New York: Bantam Books, 1974.

(Brief but concise information on over 500 herbs. Includes both plant identification as well as dosage amounts and plant properties. Excellent reference guide for anyone who is interested in herbs).

Malstrom, Stan, N.D., M.T. *Roots of Disease* (The Tree of Knowledge Book Series, Volume I). Orem, Utah: BiWorld Publishers Inc., 1979.

————. *Herbal Remedies for Common Diseases* (The Tree of Knowledge Book Series, Volume III). Orem, Utah: BiWorld Publishers Inc., 1979.

————. *Natural First Aid* (The Tree of Knowledge Book Series, Volume V). Orem, Utah: BiWorld Publishers Inc., 1979.

————. *Natural Treatment for Childhood Diseases* (The Tree of Knowledge Book Series, Volume VI). Orem, Utah: BiWorld Publishers Inc., 1979.

————. *Natural Approach to Female Problems* (The Tree of Knowledge Book Series, Volume III). Orem, Utah: BiWorld Publishers Inc., 1982.

(A comprehensive series of pamphlets that introduces the natural approach to medicine in a clear and concise manner. Common sense advice in an easy-to-read format).

Mabey, Richard, et al. *The New Age Herbalist.* New York: Macmillan Publishing Company, 1988.

(Great color photos of plants as well as chapters of information on using herbs for medicine, beauty and gardening highlight this book which suits both the student and practitioner).

Metcalfe, Joannah. *Herbs and Aromatherapy.* New York: Penguin Books, 1989.

(A handy guide to pure essential oils with easy-to-read descriptions of each oil and what it can do).

Mindell, Earl, R.Ph., Ph.D. *Earl Mindell's Herb Bible.* New York: Simon & Schuster, 1992.

(Concise information on over 100 herbs from around the world. Good quick reference guide for both the student and practitioner).

Moore, Michael. *Medicinal Plants of the Mountain West.* Santa Fe, New Mexico: The Museum of New Mexico Press, 1979.

(Dedicated exclusively to herbs which grow in the western part of the United States, Moore covers over 100 plants, their medicinal use, where to find them and the best method for gathering them).

Mowrey, Daniel B., Ph.D. *The Scientific Validation of Herbal Medicine.* New Canaan, Connecticut: Keats Publishing, Inc., 1986.

(As the title says, this book provides detailed scientific information and cold hard facts about herbs and their proven medicinal uses. Great for the practitioner who is looking to "validate" an herb).

Nuzzi, Debra, M.H. *Pocket Herbal Reference Guide.* Freedom, California: Crossing Press, 1992.

(A handy, portable reference guide chock full of herbal formulas).

Ody, Penelope. *The Complete Medicinal Herbal.* New York: Dorling Kindersley, Inc., 1993.

(Outstanding color photos and layout highlight this reference guide. Ody spotlights over 80 herbs, visually showing their various medicinal forms and briefly describing the healing properties. Wonderful book for both student and practitioner).

Ojeda, Linda. *Menopause Without Medicine.* Alameda, California: Hunter House, 1992.

(Alternative approach to "the change" without the usual drug promotion).

Olsen, Cynthia B. *Australian Tea Tree Oil Guide.* Fountain Hills, Arizona: Kali Press, 1991.

(Everything you ever wanted to know about tea tree oil is in this 68 page book. Olsen also includes clinical data to back up her facts).

Olshevsky, Moshe, et al. *The Manual of Natural Therapy.* New York: Citadel Press, 1993.

(Comprehensive guide to common ailments which focuses on the body as a whole. The book gives not only herbal information but also homeopathy, aromatherapy, acupuncture, reflexology and even autosuggestion affirmations. Great reference guide for those already familiar with alternative medicine).

Rector-Page, Linda, N.D., Ph.D. *How to Be Your Own Herbal Pharmacist.* Sonora, California: Crystal Star Herbs, 1991.

(Chock full of herbal formulas, this book is geared toward those who have a firm grasp on herbs and how to use them).

Royal, Penny C. *Herbally Yours.* Hurricane, Utah: Sound Nutrition, 1992 (38th printing).

(A quick and easy guide for both student and practitioner. Some of the herbal information is rather brief but the book works well as a companion piece to other reference materials).

Schar, Douglas. *Thirty Plants That Can Save Your Life*. Washington, D.C.: Elliott & Clark Publishing, 1993.

(Like the man says, here are 30 in-depth chapters on 30 plants that could save your life or at least improve your chances of feeling better).

Shook, Dr. Edward E. *Elementary Treatise in Herbology*. Banning, California: Enos Publishing Co., 1993 (5th printing).

(Required reading in many beginning herb courses. The book is a verbatim, unedited reproduction of the looseleaf mimeograph lessons used by Dr. Shook during his post World War II herb classes. Excellent for beginning students).

Tenney, Louise, M.H. *Health Handbook*. Provo, Utah: Woodland Books, 1987.

(Excellent pocket guide to herbs, nutrition, vitamins, minerals and amino acids. Both student and practitioner will value the information).

Theiss, Barbara & Peter. *The Family Herbal*. Rochester, Vermont: Healing Arts Press, 1989 (First edition).

(Great common-sense information on many herbs by a husband and wife who use plants in their daily lives. Also, excellent color photos of how to prepare everything from teas to poultices).

Thomas, Lalitha. *10 Essential Herbs*. Prescott, Arizona:: Hohm Press, 1992.

(A fantastic book for both student and practitioner. Thomas uses wit and personal experience to outline the 10 healing herbs she feels everyone needs in their kitchen cupboard. Her theory is that with these 10 herbs, you can take care of just about any ailment).

Tisserand, Maggie. *Aromatherapy For Women*. Rochester, Vermont: Healing Arts Press, 1988.

(Great introduction to the practical use of pure essential oils. From personal experience, Tisserand gives you a sense that the world would be a better place if we learned how to use essential oils).

Tisserand, Robert B. *The Art of Aromatherapy*. Rochester, Vermont: Healing Arts Press, 1977.

(Tisserand gives detailed information on 28 essential oils as well as in-depth information on the history, use and importance of plant-based medicine).

Treben, Maria. *Health From God's Garden.* Rochester, Vermont: Healing Arts Press, 1988.

(Treben's second book outlines uses for 35 plants. Her herbal wisdom comes from years of practicing what she preaches).

Treben, Maria. *Health Through God's Pharmacy.* Austria: Wilhelm Ennsthaler Publishing, 1980.

(Treben's first book outlines 30 herbs which she feels hold the healing answer to every ailment known to mankind. She is not afraid to say an herb "cures" even the most seemingly "incurable" health problem).

Wildwood, Christine. *Holistic Aromatherapy.* London: Thorsons, 1992.

(Wildwood gives good information on 25 essential oils, including their practical application and emotional use. She also includes an excellent ailment/oil cross reference guide).

Weiss, Gaea & Shandor. *Growing & Using The Healing Herbs.* Pennsylvania: Rodale Press, 1985.

(Good reference book for cultivating, drying and preparing medicinal plants. Includes brief information on the plant's healing properties as well as a few formulas. Both student and practitioner can benefit from the information).

INDEX

Acne 19, 38, 50, 99
Adrenal glands 108, 109
AIDS 138
Alcohol
  to decrease interest 94
Alertness 120
Allantoin 41
Allergies 109, 115
Allicin 74
Allium sativum 73
American ginseng 86, 88
Anemia 48, 129
Angelica sinensis 52
Anger 36
Anthemis nobilis 35
Antibiotic (natural) 27, 60, 73, 77, 93
Antibiotics 161
Anxiety 35, 99, 137
Aphrodisiac 91
Appetite (stimulating) 26, 36, 93
Arnica Montana 11
Arnica (homeopathic) 12-13, 169
Arnica (herb) 11-14, 152 (bath)
Arthritis 33, 62, 66, 83, 93, 100, 109-
  110, 114, 136, 142
Asthma 109, 114
Athlete's foot 157
Auto immune diseases 63
Azulene 39
Backache 22, 33, 39, 66
  from menstrual pain 54
Baldness 144
Baths, herbal,
  "Aching-Overworked bath" 152
  Arnica 14
  babies and, 153
  Cayenne 149
  Chamomile 149
  Comfrey 150
  children and, 153
  Eucalyptus 150
  essential oils 148-149
  Ginger 150
  Lavender 151, 153
  "Meditation Bath" 153
  muslin sack 149
  Mustard 151
  oil extraction 148
  Peppermint 151
  Rosemary 152

  tea 147-148
  Thyme 152
Bed wetting 138
Bedsores 17, 45
Bee stings, see Stings
Bladder (infection) 113
Bleeding 18, 30
Blister 63, 104-105, 127, 139
Bloating 54
Blood poisoning 61, 127
Blood pressure 31, 53, 74, 131
Blood purifier 19, 53, 61
Blood sugar 31, 90
Blood clots 30
Blue chamomile 38-40
Boils 94
Bones
  broken 42, 44
Bowel (restoring) 21
Brain 53, 99
Breast cancer
  estrogen-dependent 95
Breath freshener 98, 114
Bronchial congestion 42, 66, 70, 105,
  108
Bronchitis 26, 70
Bruising 12, 13, 133
Buchu 113
Burn Formula (Dr. Christopher's) 44
Burns 16, 39, 42, 44-45, 67, 104, 120,
  133, 136, 144
Calendula officinalis 15
Calendula (herb) 15-19
Candida 119
Canker sores 17
Capsicum frutescens 28
Cascara Sagrada (herb) 20-23
Catnip (herb) 24-27
Cayenne (herb) 28-34, 60, 83, 94, 149
  (bath), 169
  capsules 33-34
Cedarwood chips (bath) 153
Cellulite 100
Chamomile (herb) 35-40, 96, 149
  (bath), 169
Chamomilla (homeopathic) 40
Chapped lips 17
Chinese ginseng, see *Panax ginseng*
"Chitten Bark" 21
Cholesterol (lowering) 31, 74, 89

Christopher, John R. 2, 44-45, 131
Chronic conditions 163
Circulation 30, 80, 106
Clark's Rule 162
Cloves (bath) 153
Cockroach repellent 71
Coffee substitute 49
Cold sore 17, 63, 105, 119
Colds 26, 32, 50, 59, 64-65, 69, 74, 76, 82, 84, 106, 130-131, 142
  childhood 25
Colic 25, 36-37
Colitis 18, 23
Coltsfoot (foot bath) 156
Comfrey (herb) 41-46, 150 (bath), 152 (bath), 169
Conjunctivitis 66-67
Constipation 20
Cough 99, 105, 107-108, 124
Crying (infant) 105
Cuts 27, 77, 125
Cystitis 37
Dandelion (herb) 47-51
Dandruff 144
Dang gui, see Dong quai
Decoction 184-185
Deodorizer, room 100
Depression 99, 103, 106, 137
  contraindicated with Hops 95
Diabetes 32, 115, 155
Diaper rash, see Rashes
Diarrhea 26, 83, 130
Digestion 26, 36, 80, 83, 114, 119
Diuretic 48, 93, 97, 113
  "external" 99
Dizziness 105, 119
Dog bites 125
Dong gway, see Dong quai
Dong quai (herb) 52-57
Ear mites 77
Earache 65, 71
Echinacea (herb) 58-63
Echinacea angustifolia 58
Eczema 16, 38, 50, 100, 144
Edema 98
Elder (herb) 64-67
Elder flower/Peppermint 64-66
Eleutherococcus senticosus 86
Endocrine glands 89
Epsom salt (foot bath) 156
Essential oils,
  Blue Chamomile 38-40
  Eucalyptus 68-72, 150 (bath), 169
  German Chamomile, see Blue Chamomile
  Juniper 99-100
  Lavender 104-106, 151, 153, 169
  Parsley 115
  Peppermint 120-122, 151, 170
  Roman Chamomile 38-39
  Rosemary 152
  Thyme 152

Estrogen Replacement Therapy 55-56
Eucalyptus globulus 68
Eucalyptus 68-72
Extract 185
Fainting 105, 119
Fatigue 89, 103
Fatigue 22
Fever 26, 69, 70-71, 80, 106, 142
  baby's 25
  hot and dry 64
Fibroid cysts 57
First aid kit (herbal) 168-170
Flax seed oil 136
Fleas 71-72, 77
Flies 77, 104
Flu, see Colds
Fomentation 187-188
Foot baths, (herbal), 154-158
  Arnica 14
  Cayenne & Ginger 156
  Coltsfoot 156
  Epsom salt 156
  Horsetail 157
  Parsley 157
  Tea tree oil 157
  White Willow 158
Freckles 67
Frostbite 155
Gallbladder 48, 50
Garlic (herb) 32, 60, 73-79
  foot poultice 78
Gas 93, 114, 119
Ginger 80-85, 150 (bath), 152 (bath), 169
Ginseng 86-91
Ginseng adulteration 90-91
Glycyrrhiza glabra 107
Gout 49
Green hellebore (plant) 124
Gums (infected) 98
Hangover 105
Hay fever 66, 109
Headaches 22, 69, 81, 83, 105, 117, 140
  migraine 39, 105
  stress 82
Heart 31
Heart attack 31
Hemlock (herb) 115
Hemorrhoids 23, 45-46
Hepatitis 22
Herbal spray 193
Herpes simplex 119
HIV 138
Hops 92-96
  pillow 95
Hormones 110
  balancing 52
Horsetail (foot bath) 157
Humulus lupulus 92
Hyperactivity 94
Hypericum (homeopathic) 137

Hypericum perforatum 133
Hypoglycemia 33
Hysterectomy (post care) 110
Immune system 59, 74, 89, 99, 103-104
Infections 74-75, 104
  bladder 143
  sinus 70, 75
  staph 60
  toenail 157
Inflammation 12, 16, 39, 67, 94, 108, 134, 142
  gastric 143
  nail bed 18
Infusion 184
Inhalation, steam 192-193
Insect bites 14, 38, 98, 105, 115
Insomnia 53, 103
Intestinal flora (rebuilding) 38
Intestine 42
Japanese ginseng, see *Panax ginseng*
Jaundice 22
Juniper 97-101, 113
Juniperus communis 97
Kidneys 48
Korean ginseng, see *Panax ginseng*
Lavender 102-106, 151 (bath)
  sachets 103
Lavendula officinalis 102
Laxatives 20-21, 36, 53
Leg cramps 54, 132
Leucorrhea 104
Licorice (herb) 56, 61, 107-111, 169
Liniments 187
  Cayenne 33
Liver
  cirrhosis 48
  cleanser 19, 22, 48, 114, 131
  inflamed 51
  "organ of emotion" 51
Lung congestion 125
Lupus 63
Lymph glands 61
MAO inhibitor 137
Matricaria chamomilla 35
Memory 89
Menopause 53, 55-56, 137
Menstruation 18, 53-55
  cramps 26, 37, 100, 106, 114, 154
  promoting 26, 37, 55, 100, 113
  reducing 18, 119, 130
  regulating 18, 37, 53
Mentha piperita 117
Miscarriage (prevention) 129
Mononucleosis 61
Morning sickness 81, 83, 84
Moroccan chamomile, see Blue
  chamomile
Mosquito repellent 71, 121
Moth repellent 103
Mother's milk
  increasing 129

  reducing 115, 119
Motion sickness 81, 83, 84
Mustard (herb), 151 (bath)
Myrrh (bath) 153
Nausea 81, 83, 84
Neck (stiff) 82
Negative emotions 99
Nepeta cataria 24
Nervous exhaustion 103
Nervous system 39
Nervous tension 99
Neuralgia 66, 106, 134, 136
Nightmares, prevention of 105
Nipples (sore from nursing) 16
Oils (extracted) 190-192
  Arnica 136
  Calendula 18, 134
  Chamomile 38
  Cayenne 33
  Garlic 77, 169
  Lavender 104, 151
  Peppermint 104
  Rosemary 152
  St. John's Wort 134-136
  Thyme 152
Ointments/Salves 188-190
  Arnica 13, 14
  Calendula 16-17, 134, 135, 169
  Cayenne 33
  Comfrey 45
  Echinacea 61, 63
  Elder 67
  Plantain 126-127
Oshá (herb) 60, 61
Pain 80, 83, 142
  back 154
  coccyx 136
  joint 22, 33, 38-39, 67, 81, 82
  muscle 39, 71, 81, 82
  spine 81, 136
Panax quinquefolius 86
Panax ginseng 86, 88, 90
Parsley 112-116
  foot bath 157
Pelvic discomfort 154
Peppermint (herb) 117-122, 151 (bath), 170
Pesticide (natural) 77
Petroselinum sativum 112
Photosensitivity 138
Phytosterols 56
Pimple 105
Plantago lanceolata 123
Plantago major 123
Plantain 123-127
  cough syrup 124
PMS 50, 53, 55, 99, 103, 106, 137
Pneumonia 76
Poison ivy/oak 121, 126
Poisoning
  heavy metal 72
  lead 72

Postpartum bleeding 129
Poultice 188
Pregnancy
  tonic 128-129
  warning 8, 19, 33, 40, 56, 67, 78,
  85, 90, 100, 106, 111, 115, 121-
  122, 128, 144
Prostate
  congestion 155
  enlarged 98, 113
Prozac 138
Pseudo ginseng 88
Pyrrolizidine alkaloids 42
Radiation therapy 62
Ragweed (allergy) 40
Rashes 50, 124, 127
  diaper 18
Recuperation 114, 131
Red Raspberry 128-132, 170
Red Turkey Oil 148
Respiratory 66, 69, 70, 76, 99
Reye's Syndrome 144
Rhamnus purshiana 20
Rheumatism 66, 93, 100, 106, 114,
  142
Rubus idaeus 128
Rubus strigosus 128
Sage (bath) 153
Salix alba 140
Sambucus nigra 64
Sandalwood (bath) 153
Sarsaparilla (herb) 89
Scabs 17
Scars (prevention of) 16, 45
Sciatica 66, 93, 100, 106
Scrapes 16, 27, 38, 104, 120
Sedative 25, 53
Sex
  to decrease interest 94, 102, 145
Shingles 106
Shock 30, 105
Siberian ginseng 86, 88-89
Sinus congestion 69, 114, 120
Skin 67
  dry, cracked 17
  eruptions 127
  tonic 50
  ulcers 45, 94, 126, 144
Snake bite 61-62, 98
Spider bites
  Black widow 29
Sprains 14, 33, 38, 42, 44
Spray, herbal 193
"Spring Tonic" 131
St. John's Wort 133-139
Staph infections, see Infections

Steam inhalation 192-193
Stinging nettle (herb), antidote to 126
Stings 115, 125
  bee 29-30, 98, 105
  wasp 89, 105, 125-126
Strep throat 60-61, 76
Stress 88-89
Stretch marks 106
Sty 37
Sunburn 103
Suspicion, countering feeling of 106
Sweaty feet 157, 158
Symphytum officinale 41
Symphytum (tincture) 42-43
Symphytum (homeopathic tablets) 43-
  44
Syrup 186-187
Tang kwei, see Dong quai
Tang kuei, see Dong quai
Taraxacum officinale 47
Tea tree oil (foot bath) 157
Tendons (torn) 42
Throat
  sore 32, 69-70
  strep, see strep throat
Ticks 77, 105
Tinctures 185-186
  Arnica 13-14, 169
  Calendula 17-18, 134, 169
  Comfrey 42-43
  Echinacea 59-61, 62, 169
  Elder 66
  Hops 94
  Hypericum (St. John's Wort) 134-
  135, 136
TMJ 14
Toothache 93
Ulcer 18, 23, 32, 37, 110
Urination
  burning 98
Uva ursi 113
Varicose veins 17, 31
Vertigo 84
Viruses 59-60
Warts 47
Wasp stings, see Stings
Weight loss 50
White Willow (herb) 140-145, 158
  (foot bath), 170
Wildcrafting 166
Withdrawal (drugs & alcohol) 94
Worms (pets) 77
Wounds 42, 45, 61, 63, 124, 125, 126
  133, 134, 143-144
Zingiber officinale 80